Public Health Nursing

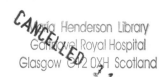

Henderson Library
Gartnavel Royal Hospital
Glasgow G12 0XH Scotland

GARTNAVEL ROYAL HOSPITAL

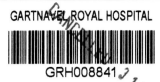

GRH008841

Public Health Nursing

A Textbook for Health Visitors, School Nurses and Occupational Health Nurses

Edited by

Greta Thornbory

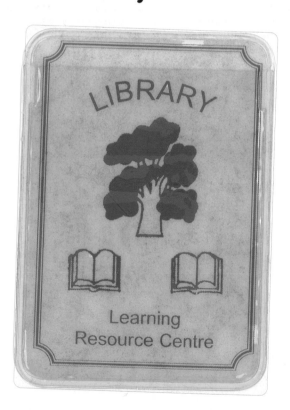

WILEY-BLACKWELL

A John Wiley & Sons, Ltd., Publication

This edition first published 2009
© 2009 Blackwell Publishing Ltd

Blackwell Publishing was acquired by John Wiley & Sons in February 2007. Blackwell's publishing programme has been merged with Wiley's global Scientific, Technical, and Medical business to form Wiley-Blackwell.

Registered office
John Wiley & Sons Ltd, The Atrium, Southern Gate, Chichester, West Sussex, PO19 8SQ, United Kingdom

Editorial offices
9600 Garsington Road, Oxford, OX4 2DQ, United Kingdom
2121 State Avenue, Ames, Iowa 50014-8300, USA

For details of our global editorial offices, for customer services and for information about how to apply for permission to reuse the copyright material in this book please see our website at www.wiley.com/wiley-blackwell.

The right of the author to be identified as the author of this work has been asserted in accordance with the Copyright, Designs and Patents Act 1988.

All rights reserved. No part of this publication may be reproduced, stored in a retrieval system, or transmitted, in any form or by any means, electronic, mechanical, photocopying, recording or otherwise, except as permitted by the UK Copyright, Designs and Patents Act 1988, without the prior permission of the publisher.

Wiley also publishes its books in a variety of electronic formats. Some content that appears in print may not be available in electronic books.

Designations used by companies to distinguish their products are often claimed as trademarks. All brand names and product names used in this book are trade names, service marks, trademarks or registered trademarks of their respective owners. The publisher is not associated with any product or vendor mentioned in this book. This publication is designed to provide accurate and authoritative information in regard to the subject matter covered. It is sold on the understanding that the publisher is not engaged in rendering professional services. If professional advice or other expert assistance is required, the services of a competent professional should be sought.

Library of Congress Cataloging-in-Publication Data

Public health nursing : a textbook for health visitors, school nurses, and occupational health nurses/edited by Greta Thornbory.
        p. ; cm.
   Includes bibliographical references and index.
   ISBN 978-1-4051-8007-8 (pbk. : alk. paper)   1. Public health nursing—Textbooks.
I. Thornbory, Greta.
   [DNLM: 1. Public Health Nursing—Great Britain. WY 108 P9762 2009]

   RT97.P838 2009
   610.73′4—dc22

                                                                    2009009963

A catalogue record for this book is available from the British Library.

Set in 9/12.5 pt Interstate Light by Aptara® Inc., New Delhi, India
Printed and bound in Malaysia by KHL Printing Co Sdn Bhd

1   2009

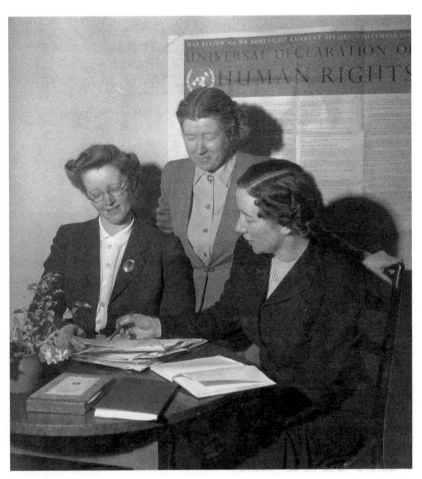

The Royal College of Nursing Public Health Department 1952. (Reproduced by permission of RCN Archives)

Maria Henderson Library
Gartnavel Royal Hospital
Glasgow G12 0XH Scotland

Contents

Contributors

Gillian Coverdale, MPH, BSc (Hons), RGN, SCPHN School Nursing, Cert Ed
Senior Lecturer/Course Leader (Specialist Community Public Health
Nursing – School Nursing), Leeds Metropolitan University

*Rebecca Elliott, M Med Sci Primary and Community Care, BSc (Hons) OH, RGN,
SCPHN OH, PGCE*
Senior Lecturer/Course Leader, BSc (Hons), PGDip/MSc Specialist
Community Public Health Nursing (Occupational Health), Leeds Metropolitan
University

Cécile Knai, MPH, PhD
Research Fellow in Public Health, Health Services Research Unit, London
School of Hygiene & Tropical Medicine

Faith Muir, MA (Ed), BA (Hons), SCPHN (HV), RGN, Dip Child Protection, CPT
Senior Lecturer, Specialist Community Public Health Nursing (Health
Visiting)/Masters of Public Health, University of Wolverhampton

Paul Reynolds, MA (Ed), BSc (Hons), RGN, SCPHN (HV), Practice Teacher
Senior Lecturer, Pathway Leader Specialist Community Public Health
Nursing (Health Visiting), University of Wolverhampton

*Sarah Sherwin, MA (Ed), BSc (Hons), RGN, SCPHN School Nursing, Diploma
Health Education, Practice Teacher*
Senior Lecturer and Course Leader for School Nursing, School of Health,
University of Wolverhampton

Mary Smith, MSc Child Health, LLM, BA, RGN, RM, SCPHN (HV), PGCE (FE)
Senior Lecturer, University of Glamorgan, Pontypridd, Course Leader for
Specialist Community Public Health Nursing (Health Visiting, School Nursing
and Occupational Health Nursing)

Greta Thornbory, TD, MSc OH, RGN, SCPHN OH, Dip N OH, PGCEA, CMIOSH
Occupational Health and Educational Consultant, previously Senior Lecturer
and Programme Director of both OH and CPD, Institute of Advanced Nursing
Education, Royal College of Nursing

Contributors

Gillian Abercrombie, MPH, BA, (Hons), RGN, SCPHN School Nursing, Cert Ed
Senior Collarer Course Leader (Specialist Community Public Health
Nursing), School Nursing, Leeds Metropolitan University

Rebecca Elliott, RN and Sch Primary and Community Care DipHVisor, DipHVisor
SCPHN OH, PGCE
Senior Lecturer/Course Leader, PGC (Hons), PGDip, MSc, Specialist
Community Public Health Nursing (Occupational Health), Leeds Metropolitan
University

Clare Bale, MPH, PhD
Research Fellow in Public Health, Health Sciences Research Unit, London
School of Hygiene & Tropical Medicine

Ruth Mann, MA (Ed), BA (Hons), SCPHN (HV), RGN, Dip Child Protection, CMT
Senior Lecturer, Specialist Community Public Health Nursing (Health
Visiting), Faculty of Health, University of Wolverhampton

Paul Reynolds, MA, PhD, BSc (Hons), RMN, SCPHN (HV), Practice Teacher
Senior Lecturer Pathway Leader, Specialist Community Public Health
Nursing (Health Visiting), University of Wolverhampton

Sadie Shorter, MA (Ed), PGC (Prof), RGN, SCPHN School Nursing, Diploma
Health Education, Practice Teacher
Senior Lecturer and Course Leader for School Nursing, School of Health,
University of Wolverhampton

Ruth Smith, MSc, Dip Health, LLM, BA, RGN, RM, SCPHN (Health Visiting)
Senior Lecturer University of Glamorgan, PgDip, BSc, Course Leader for
Specialist Community Public Health Nursing (Health Visiting, School Nursing
and Occupational Health Nursing)

Greta Thornbory, TD, MSc OH, RGN, SCPHN OH, Dip NEBOSH, PGCEA, FAOHP
Occupational Health and Educational Consultant, previously Senior Lecturer
and Programme Director of both OH and CPD, Institute of Advanced Nursing
Education, Royal College of Nursing

Forewords

Health Visiting

Throughout the history of health visiting, public health has been the underpin-ning aspect of the work of health visitors. This book articulates the changing role of health visitors in providing a dynamic service whilst engaging in in-novative ways to tackle the complex needs of society today. The search for health needs have been identified by professional organisations as an impor-tant aspect of health visiting practice. The authors clearly define health within a public health dimension, whilst detailing the concept of health promotion as the process, which facilitates change and allows the health visitor to deliver a service, which acknowledges the demands of a multifarious approach.

The phenomenon of social capital as pivotal to public health and health policy gives the reader insight into the challenges of health visiting in an ever-changing society. The four principles of health visiting are clearly identified as central to health visiting practice. Although it is acknowledged in current legislation there is still much to achieve as far as public health is concerned, the authors state that the role of health visiting is less clear and health visitor numbers are reducing allowing them less time to focus on early intervention in health issues.

This book focuses on the importance of health visitors being politically aware in order to tackle the effect of poverty especially on the development of children. The authors emphasise the importance of community profiling which has long been a desirable attribute of health visiting activities.

This book also provides a sound underpinning for student health visitors as well as being reminders of the role health visitors have in public health to those health visitors and their managers in practice. The authors have captured the essential components of public health practice and the role that health visitors can play.

Dr Ingrid Callwood
Head of Division, Community Health, University of Wolverhampton

School Nursing

In the century since school nursing began, understanding of child development, education and nursing skills have been transformed. Chapter 5 maps developments in both school environments and the National Health Service. The current health of the school-aged population predicts of adult health for decades ahead – and economic well-being, and social stability. The new Department for Children, Schools and Families (DCSF) recognises this *pervasive* public health role of school nurses. The DCSF values school nursing expertise in delivering strategies for population health because of its unique impact on outcomes for children. This impact can be seen both in school and across wider community settings. Society's response to illness, adversity or abuse for individual children mirrors its *deepest* values. While enlightened policies such as the Special Educational Needs and Disability Act 2001 reflected noble aims, a 2008 survey for *Every Disabled Child Matters* revealed not one Primary Care Trust could quantify their spend on services for disabled children. England produced model *specialist* services for mental illness in young people, but now at the community level English adolescents have the worst mental well-being in the Western World. I discussed these concerns with the Children's Commissioner for England (around giving *11 Million* children a 'voice'): he emphasised the folly of the media 'demonising' teenagers. School nurses can work alongside young people in a responsive and accountable way that anticipates transitions and their growing capacity for responsibility. School nursing evolved unique *ethical* foundations that encompass 'vulnerable' individuals, groups of children and networks of parents or professionals. Those ethics underpin the duty of care described here.

Nurses work for the school-aged population within teams, within a variety of settings. Chapter 6 illustrates the standards for Specialist Community Public Health Nursing, relating this nurse to the wider school health service. Consultation with young people and a capacity to advocate for children based on evidence of their health needs are *key* skills to nurture. When professional training and development was going through a period of neglect concerns were often expressed about the poor evidence base for practice and the paucity of efforts to explain school nursing to other professions, especially general practitioners or service commissioners. Clear practical examples of school health expertise are provided here, e.g. for the epidemic of obesity sweeping the UK. The promotion of 'positive mental health' gives a good grounding for coming initiatives like *Targeted Mental Health in Schools*. These chapters foresee the professional need to enhance 'collaborative working' across all the agencies involved in young people's well-being. SCPHNs have been at the forefront of recent developments to *integrate* services for every child (ages 0-19) and the professional bodies have seized this challenge to combine innovation with evidence-based practice. The example given of raised standards in personal, social and health education, through an effective collaboration between school nurses and both primary and secondary school teachers, shows us all the way ahead.

Woody Caan
Professor of Public Health, Department of Child & Family Health,
Anglia Ruskin University, Cambridge

Occupational Health Nursing

The contribution of occupational health (OH) nurses to public health is not new as they have promoted health and practiced at a strategic level for many years. Their contemporary public health role is recognised by the Nursing and Midwifery Council (NMC) as those holding an NMC-validated qualification in OH nursing can register as specialist community public health nurses.

OH nurses by definition practice with a specific client group – the workforce. They undertake a proactive role in reducing health inequalities amongst that population. These specialists are involved in policy development and undertake a population-based approach rather than merely providing care to individuals, these are important elements of public health practice.

The workforce is a captive audience for a range of health-promoting activities and never before has the OH nurse's contribution to public health been higher profile. Dame Carol Black's recent review of the health of Britain's working-age population, *Working for a Healthier Tomorrow*, has been a particular influence on public health and on OH nursing practice in particular. Black's review emphasises the premise that promoting, improving and maintaining the health of the working-age population makes a significant contribution to the nation's economic growth and social justice.

An experienced OH nurse educationalist and consultant has edited this book which provides a succinct overview of a workplace-focused public health strategy. It explores the four levels of primordial, primary, secondary and tertiary prevention linking these to contemporary OHN practice and highlights the role of the OHN in advising and supporting employers in ensuring a healthy and productive workforce. It is written in such a way that nurses new to OH nursing as well as those with more experience will benefit from its exploration of the role and function of the OHN within a multidisciplinary team.

Anne Harriss
Reader in Educational Development and Course Director,
Specialist Community Public Health Nursing (Occupational Health)
Programmes,
London South Bank University

Preface

Public health (PH) nursing is not a new nursing discipline, but with the advent of the Nursing and Midwifery Council pulling together the nursing disciplines that work in the field of public health it has been necessary to address the issue with a textbook on the subject. Specialist education and training is required to prepare the qualified nurse to undertake PH nursing work as there is evidence that PH is currently taking centre stage in the challenge to improve the population's health and nursing should be playing an active part.

This book is a basic text aimed at those nurses new to the PH arena and who are undertaking specialist education and training. It is written by relevant experts in the field and the three main specialties of PH nursing, health visitors, who care for families and children up to five; school nurses, who care for the school-aged child and occupational health nurses, who care for the health and well-being of people at work. It does not aim to be all embracing of each discipline, it is designed to be read in conjunction with each discipline's specialist textbooks and the references and resources given in the book should act as pointers for further more in-depth reading and information.

One of the book's main aims is to show the diversity of each discipline and how they each address PH in vastly different ways according to the needs of their relevant population. The book starts by exploring the term *public health* and then how it relates to nursing. The chapters that follow then address each discipline in turn and conclude with a chapter on the all-important continuing professional development.

Greta Thornbory

Acknowledgements

I would like to thank the following people for their contributions, help, advice and support in writing this book: All the chapter contributors for their endless patience and for being on time; Rachel Coombs at Wiley-Blackwell for her advice and support with this project; Dr Stuart Whitaker who kindly undertook the job of critical reader; Anne Harriss and Robert Dunn who have given me endless support; All the PH practitioners who have provided examples from practice and they include: Lee Bromwich, Caroline Forrest, Sharon George, Sue Jones, Cassie Parsons, Anne Roberts, Angie Waldron, Penny Wilson, Denize Bainbridge, Christina Butterworth, Jenny Mason, Sandra Neylon, Sue Gee and Gillian Eastwood.

Finally, to Sue Hincliffe who encouraged me on the road to writing.

Greta Thornbory

Abbreviations

ACAS	Advisory, Conciliation and Arbitration Service
AOHNE	Association of Occupational Health Nurse Educators
AOHNP	Association of Occupational Health Nurse Practitioners
BOHS	British Occupational Hygiene Society
CAMHS	Child and Adolescent Mental Health Services
CBI	Confederation of British Industry
CDC	Centre for Disease Control and Prevention
CETHV	Council for the Education and Training of Health Visitors
CHPP	Child Health Promotion Programme
CIPD	Chartered Institute of Personnel and Development
CPD	Continuing Professional Development
CPHVA	Community Practitioners and Health Visitors Association
CTHV	Council for the Training of Health Visitors
DDA	Disability Discrimination Act 2005
DEA	Disabled Employment Advisor
DPA	Data Protection Act 1998
DSE	Display Screen Equipment (previously VDU or visual display unit)
EAP	Employee Assistance Programme
EEF	Engineering Employers Federation
ELCI	Employers Liability Compulsory Insurance
EU	European Union
FAO	United Nations' Food and Agriculture Organization
GMC	General Medical Council
GP	General Practitioner
HASAWA	Health and Safety at Work (etc.) Act 1974
HPC	Health Professions Council
HPV	Human Papilloma Virus
HR	Human Resources
HSE	Health and Safety Executive
HV	Health Visitor
ILO	International Labor Organization
IOSH	Institute of Occupational Safety and Health
LEA	Local Education Authority
LLM	Master of Laws
MHSW	Management of Health and Safety at Work Regulations 1999
MMR	Measles, Mumps and Rubella

MSDs	Musculoskeletal Disorders
NATHNAC	National Travel Health Network and Centre
NAW	National Assembly for Wales
NFSHE	National Forum for School Health Educators
NHS	National Health Service
NMC	Nursing and Midwifery Council
OFSTED	Office for Standards in Education
OH	Occupational Health
OHN	Occupational Health Nurse
OM	Occupational Medicine
PCT	Primary Care Trust
PGCE	Post Graduate Certificate of Education
PGCEA	Post Graduate Certificate of Education of Adults
PH	Public Health
PSA	Public Sector Agreement
PSHE	Personal, Social and Health Education
RCN	Royal College of Nursing
RTWI	Return to Work Interviews
SAPHNA	School and Public Health Nurses Association
SCPHN	Specialist Community Public Health Nurses
SMEs	Small- and Medium-Sized Enterprises
SNs	School Nurses
UKCC	United Kingdom Central Council
UKSC	United Kingdom Standing Conference
VRA	Vocational Rehabilitation Association
WHO	World Health Organization

Chapter 1
What Is Public Health?

Cécile Knai

Learning objectives

After reading this chapter you will be able to:

- Discuss the meaning of public health
- Describe the changing approaches to public health over time
- Discuss some of the current debates within public health
- Comment on some of the implications of health practitioners

Introduction

This chapter attempts to answer the question 'What is public health?' and at one level, the answer is simple and straightforward: public health aims at preventing health problems before they occur and focuses on populations rather than on individuals. As we will see in the chapter, there are different ways of going about this task. The more convenient linear, two-dimensional way holds that there is a cause and there is a disease, and to address the disease one needs to address the cause. According to this line of thought, disease is brought about by specific aetiological agents which affect the body's structure and function, with illness a separate 'subjective experience of dysfunction' [1]. This biomedical model has been argued as being narrow: the reality is that achieving public health is a complex task with an ill-defined scope. This is not for lack of effort on behalf of public health practitioners. Indeed, as discussed below, an enormous amount of effort and debate and political commitment have converged over time so that the field of public health is a field in its own right, with educational and professional specialisations. The approach to health has shifted from a relatively narrow approach to a broader conception of what health means, as expressed by the World Health Organization (WHO) definition which has not been amended since 1948: 'Health is a state of complete physical, mental and social well-being and not merely the absence of disease or infirmity' [2]. Moreover, the understanding of public health and the extent to which governments should intervene to support population health will vary according to the sociopolitical stance of countries [3, 4].

This chapter introduces the various meanings and applications of public health, placing it in a historical context to help the reader to understand the development of modern public health. We highlight some of the major achievements of the past century, and discuss the current challenges we face. The discussion of these challenges provides an opportunity to understand some of the underlying philosophical and practical debates in public health. Finally, we suggest some of the implications for health practitioners. Although many of these arguments are universal, this chapter mainly draws on European context and highlights the experience and development of public health in Britain.

The development of modern public health

An early definition of public health, variations of which have informed later definitions, is that of Winslow from the 1920s. Winslow proposed that public health was 'the science and art of preventing disease, prolonging life, and promoting mental and physical health and efficiency through organised community efforts for the sanitation of the environment, the control of communicable infections, the education of the individual in personal hygiene, the organisation of medical and nursing services for the early diagnosis and preventive treatment of disease, and the development of social machinery to ensure to every individual a standard of living adequate for the maintenance of health, so organising these benefits as to enable every citizen to realise his birthright of health and longevity' [5].

Although the wording is slightly dated, the meaning still holds. Importantly, it demonstrates the many overlapping disciplines comprising public health, adapted according to time and context. The modern field of public health is highly varied and encompasses many academic disciplines including the fundamental tools of epidemiology, biostatistics, health education, advocacy, policy analysis and health services management applied to various fields such as environmental health, food and nutrition, tobacco and alcohol abuse, and the health of different age groups across the life course. Increasingly, a crucial facet of public health research and practice has been to factor in as thoroughly as possible factors such as social, economic, cultural, psychological and political considerations since they characterise the diverse aspects of health risk in different ways and to different degrees of importance according to context [6].

The question of whether public health should confine itself to individual risk factors for disease or rather be increasingly concerned with the more 'upstream' sources of health (or ill health) such as employment, housing, transport, food and nutrition and global trade concerns is central to public debates and in many ways defined by the political and economic stance of those on either side of the debate. Beaglehole and Bonita [7] argue that 'the central challenge for public health practitioners is to articulate and act upon a broad definition of public health which incorporates a multidisciplinary and intersectoral approach to the underlying causes of premature death and disability'.

Origins and history of public health

Understanding the historical development of the public health movement provides perspective on current health issues and on the wider significance and impact of health interventions [8]. Writing for the journal *Public Health* in 1928, Wood notes that above and beyond the great achievements of public health in Britain, there were 'adverse circumstances still requiring attention', citing, for example, the appalling conditions in newly industrialising cities and stating that 'in the forefront I would place one of our last remaining problems of environmental hygiene, the smoke pollution of the atmosphere, with its direct and indirect effects on physical well-being' [9]. Many of the discussions of the past resonate with contemporary ones.

The ideology and concept of public health and how it is organised and implemented have undergone important changes over time. The history of public health stretches back to 'remote times' [10], by some accounts as far as the ancient Greeks [11]. The growing involvement of 'authorities' in addressing the health problems of citizens progressively increased with the approach of the modern era [10], many examples of which have been documented (read, for example, *Occupational Health and Public Health: Lessons from the Past - Challenges for the Future* [4] and *Public Health at the Crossroads: Achievements and Prospects* [11]). George Rosen's *A History of Public Health* [12] provides an in-depth account of the development of public health over time and throughout the world. For the purposes of this chapter, we focus on developments in Europe and particularly Britain and step into the history of public health at the time of industrialisation, particularly its consequences on the health of urban populations, and the debates and policy decisions it engendered.

The nineteenth century saw an increasingly systematic approach to public health, taking root throughout European countries, with considerable scientific advances and a growing consciousness of the impact of life in industrial cities on the health of populations.

In Britain the sanitary movement was launched in the 1820s, emphasising the need for government-level expertise in health [13]. It is argued that the sanitary movement was motivated and led by the work of social reformers rather than medical practitioners [11]. During his travels through Britain in the 1830s, the French political thinker Alexis de Tocqueville commented on the abject conditions of urban centres, noting that here '... humanity attains its most complete development and its most brutish; here civilization works its miracles, and here civilized man is turned back almost into a savage' [14].

During the 1840s, public health emerged as a field in its own right in Britain. A key player in the 'meshing of medicine with the moral and political economy' [15] was Edwin Chadwick. His seminal 1842 report on the sanitary conditions of the working class revealed the dangerous conditions in which labourers lived and worked [11]. This report was the first such national investigation and pointed to a number of now widely accepted phenomena about economic development, urbanisation and health within industrial urban areas [15]. Chadwick supported the principle that the people's health was a matter of public concern and thus one of the responsibilities of the state [16]. He highlighted through his report how modern circumstances could contribute to a health schism between social groups [15]. One of the conclusions of this report was that '... the various forms of epidemic, endemic, and other disease caused, or aggravated, or propagated chiefly amongst the labouring classes by atmospheric impurities produced by decomposing animal and vegetable substances, by damp and filth, and close and overcrowded dwellings prevail amongst the population in every part of the kingdom, whether dwelling in separate houses, in rural villages, in small towns, in the larger towns – as they have been found to prevail in the lowest districts of the metropolis' [17]. This document was not only a survey of the social and environmental condition of towns and cities, but in effect an act to bring together formerly isolated health and sanitary domains, and to create public health policy [15]. The subsequent Public Health Act of 1848 was a legislative attempt to impart social and health equity in Britain [11]. It was built upon the assumption that implementation of the sanitary reform would address and remove causes of illness and early death, and allow labourers to live longer and healthier lives and thus contribute to the economy [18]. Then, as now, however, the battle was to convince government that these ideas were viable, particularly in the light of the great costs related to sanitary measures [18]. It saw the establishment of the Board of Health, though reportedly unpopular and short-lived because it challenged powerful vested interests: it faced strong opposition from the medical profession and local government officials reluctant to yield to a central authority. It is reported that by the 1870s the medical profession dominated public health in Britain; this dominance continues in most European countries including the United Kingdom [11, 19].

The Public Health Act was shaped by the prevailing miasmic medical notions, or the idea that disease is associated with noxious odours, impure air and poor sanitation [15] (miasma translates as 'bad air' in Greek). This was of course subsequently refuted, as described below. But by the 1850s, as a result of the Public Health Act there were better sewers, cleaner water and streets less polluted with decaying animals and human excrement. Disease did in fact decline, providing empirical evidence for these disease theories [18]. However, at this time great scientific advances contributed to the understanding of how disease was caused and spread. It was the French microbiologist Louis Pasteur who 'dealt the final blow to [...] miasma as the cause of infectious diseases' [18]. In short, Pasteur is credited with reframing disease by demonstrating what eventually came to be known as the 'germ theory', namely, that specific microbes caused specific diseases, an unthinkable concept until then. Towards the end of the nineteenth century, the German scientist Robert Koch devised a series of proofs or criteria to establish a causal relationship between a microbe and a disease, now referred to as 'Koch's postulates', and these supported the germ theory [11, 13]. One of Chadwick's contemporaries, John Snow, was a strong supporter of the germ theory. He is credited with carrying out one of the first epidemiological study in 1854, now commonly referred to as the study of the Broad Street Pump: while investigating a local cholera epidemic in London, Snow linked all cases to a single contaminated well. He convinced authorities to remove the pump handle and the spread of the disease was rapidly reduced. Snow isolated what would eventually be identified as the bacterium responsible for cholera.

By the turn of the century there was no longer any question that certain microbes caused specific diseases, and slowly but surely major cities were building sewages systems and providing cleaner water for their inhabitants. These advances provided a solid foundation for contemporary measures for communicable diseases control and laid the scientific basis for vaccination [18, 20].

The early twentieth century saw the rise of preventive medicine, characterised by its focus on the concept of hygiene, supporting the previous developments in several ways [20]: it took into account the concept of disease vectors; it highlighted the importance of nutrition and the role of nutrient deficiencies in impairing optimal health (thus leading to the development of vitamins); and it emphasised the particular needs of 'high-risk' population groups such as schoolchildren, pregnant women and older people [21]. Advances in housing, education, road and other infrastructure enabled rapid economic progress to take place across Europe during this period and this undoubtedly did much to improve the health of those populations.

The assumption of scientific rationality where disease aetiology follows a relatively linear pathway [1] was increasingly challenged by many as failing to capture all factors pertinent to disease: broad social conditions must be addressed by all relevant sectors to bring about long-term and meaningful improvements in population health [22, 23]. These principles were supported and developed by a series of important policy commitments at the national and international level. The 1974 Lalonde Report by the Canadian Government proposed the health field concept wherein genetic predisposition, individual behaviour and lifestyle, health services and environmental circumstances all contribute to population health [24]. A focus on healthy public policy and intersectoral action was then laid out in 1978 by the WHO's 'Health for All by the Year 2000' movement [25], the key principles of which were (1) global cooperation and peace as important aspects of primary health care; (2) recognition that primary health care should be adapted to the particular circumstances of a country and the communities within it; (3) recognition that health care reflects broader social and economic development; (4) primary health care as the backbone of a nation's health strategy, with an emphasis on health promotion and disease prevention strategies; (5) achievement of equity in health status; and (6) involvement of all sectors in the promotion of health [26].

These principles were enshrined in the 1986 Ottawa Charter for Health Promotion which called for building healthy public policy, creating supportive environments, strengthening community actions, developing personal skills, reorienting health services and demonstrating commitment to health promotion [24]. The conference participants challenged the WHO and other international organisations 'to advocate the promotion of health in all appropriate forums and to support countries in setting up strategies and programmes for health promotion' [27]. These commitments continue to be renewed by WHO and are increasingly cross-disciplinary to ensure a broad enough scope of action and influence.

Moreover, the ecological approach to public health is increasingly accepted. In public health, an ecological model refers to people's interactions with their physical and sociocultural surroundings [28], incorporating many influences at multiple levels [29, 30] including biological, psychological, cultural, physical (built and natural environment) and policy [31]. Although there are ongoing debates about whether this is an appropriate approach or not, the ecological approach is supported by influential public health publications such as the WHO/FAO report Diet, Nutrition and the Prevention of Chronic Disease [32] and by the WHO Global Strategy for Diet and Physical Activity [33].

Successes and challenges in public health

The advances in public health over the past century, due in part to the convergence of scientific progress and political commitment, have improved our quality of life [34]. In 1999, the US Centre for Communicable Disease Control published a list of the twentieth century's ten greatest public health achievements [35]. These are summarised below. As noted in an article by Gray et al., these achievements are all applicable to the United Kingdom where they have significantly contributed to considerable, long-term increases in life expectancy [36, 37]:

(1) Vaccination resulted in the eradication of smallpox; elimination of polio (in the Americas); and control of measles, rubella, tetanus, diphtheria and Haemophilus influenzae type b

(2) Motor-vehicle safety led to substantial reductions in motor vehicle-related deaths due to engineering improvements in vehicles and highways, and changes in personal behaviours such as using seat belts and other safety devices, and reductions in drinking and driving

(3) Safer workplaces due to a focus on occupational health and environments led to, e.g., the control of pneumoconiosis and silicosis and a reduction in fatal occupational injuries

(4) Reduction of infectious diseases was achieved through the control of typhoid and cholera by focusing on improving water and sanitation, and the control of tuberculosis and sexually transmitted diseases (STDs) by education and the advent of antibiotics

(5) A decline in deaths from coronary heart disease and stroke was attained from changing high-risk behaviours, such as smoking cessation and blood pressure control, and improved access to early detection and treatment

(6) Safer and healthier foods contributed to nearly eliminating nutritional deficiency diseases such as rickets, goitre and pellagra, and were achieved by decreasing microbial contamination and increasing nutritional content

(7) Advances in maternal and child health came about through better hygiene and nutrition, availability of antibiotics, access to health care and technological advances in neonatal and maternal medicine

(8) Family planning contributed to improved maternal and child health and supported a more important socioeconomic role of women, reduced family size, and increased birth intervals; barrier contraceptives also reduced unwanted pregnancies and transmission of STDs

(9) Fluoridation of drinking water contributed to reducing tooth decay and tooth loss

(10) Recognition of tobacco use as a health hazard resulted in changes in social norms, reduced prevalence of tobacco smoking and mortality and morbidity from smoking-related diseases

Although these have certainly been important successes in population health due to public health strategies and the role of public health is increasingly recognised, implementation is more often than not difficult to achieve [38]. Philosophical debates continue on who holds the responsibility for action in health, as well as how best to translate scientifically independent and comparable data into effective public health policy. The following section addresses some of these challenges.

The responsibility for health

Individuals and nation states will have different understandings of how to achieve a population which benefits from 'a state of complete physical, mental and social well-being'. These differences are grounded in sociocultural and political stance. Traditionally, a more liberal group will support minimal government intervention, whereas a more socialist group may have more faith in the effects of policy. This debate is important as it is a decisive factor in the direction a government will take in addressing public health at the national level. The health status of a population will be affected by its culture, economy and social norms [3, 4]. These factors will often dictate or at least influence the extent to which public health practitioners will be successful in convincing policy- and decision-makers of the need for addressing particular determinants of ill health as broadly and comprehensively as possible.

This debate has taken several forms and has been expressed in social and political philosophies. The eighteenth- and nineteenth-century responses to this question were most powerfully formulated by philosophers and political economists who held that the free functioning of individual choice and freedom would be the best way to work in the interest of public good. The utilitarian criterion for deciding where to set the boundary between the private and the public was the notion of harm; the private was the realm in which action did not harm others [39]: 'The only purpose for which power can be rightfully exercised over any number of a civilized community, against his will, is to prevent harm to others. His own good, either physical or moral, is not a sufficient warrant [...] The only part of the conduct of anyone, for which that concerns others [...] over himself, over his own body and mind, the individual is sovereign' [40]. The notion of what constituted harm has, however, expanded, as it became increasingly clear that private actions could have public consequences. Thus, in the late nineteenth century, certain kinds of problems such as housing, health and education were no longer considered private matters and were taken into the public sphere of interest.

By the early twentieth century, proponents of a 'new liberalism' had emerged, as expressed by writers such as J. M. Keynes in Britain, to argue that a more knowledgeable form of governance was required to balance public and private claims and interests. Thus, the role of the state should be to manage the public sphere and its problems so as to address aspects of social and economic life that markets were no longer capable of solving.

The 1970s saw a revival of libertarianism with, for example, Friedrich Hayek and Milton Friedman, who argued that the attempt to use public policy to promote the public interest was flawed [41]; rather the relationship between private and public was best defined by the market and freedom of choice. John Rawls provided a strong counter-argument by considering public interests in terms of fairness and equality of opportunity, arguing that justice has to do with the distribution of outcomes in a fair way, where differences could be accepted if social and economic inequalities maximised benefits to the least advantaged [42]. Those that supported his approach considered it a key philosophical underpinning of public policy, yet those that critiqued his approach, such as Robert Nozick, suggested that justice does not have to do with fairness but with what people are entitled to [43], maintaining, as did the early libertarians, that the organisation of society through the forces of individuals and markets is the only way forward for the attainment of justice [39].

These philosophical arguments continue and are well represented within the field of public health. Where does the onus for action in population health lie? Environmental and policy changes are at the centre of the ecological approach and have been identified as the most promising strategy for bringing about population-wide improvements in diet, physical activity and other key determinants of health [31, 44–46]. Critics argue that taking an ecological approach to address disease prevention and health promotion threatens 'informed choice' through societal paternalism or 'nanny-statism'. Moreover, factors dictating the health of populations include not only behaviours and attitudes but also genetic profile and family history, factors that are not necessarily subject to modification. The example of obesity challenges this argument: the rapidity with which rates of obesity are growing in virtually all countries of Europe and the rest of the world far exceeds the speed with which genetic mutations develop. Proponents of the ecological approach to disease prevention might respond that the development of policies and regulations is not a question of challenging informed choice; rather it is a question of creating an environment conducive to increased physical activity (e.g. urban planning policies that help to increase access to parks and playgrounds) and healthy diet (e.g. food and nutrition policies that help to make fruit and vegetables affordable and available); legislating corporate conduct where there is clear conflict of interest and ethical issues (e.g. advertising soft drinks in the classroom) and a reasonable probability of negative impact on children's behaviour; and learning how to disseminate the public health message in a more sustainable, effective way. An individual who is deemed competent is ultimately responsible for his or her actions; however, these actions occur within a specific context which inevitably imparts a positive or negative influence. Vulnerable groups, such as the unborn child, children and young people, the elderly or disabled, and those with mental incapacity may need additional protections. Behavioural change is notoriously difficult to bring about in isolation from the context from which it emerges, thus making preventive strategies targeting individual change often ineffective [47, 48]. In reality, those most likely to become ill are those with the least ability to make healthy choices because of the structural, social, organisational, financial and other constraints they face, and fundamentally, behaviour is directly related to and perhaps even a result of the conditions in which they live [47, 49, 50]. Eisenberg wrote in 1977 that 'the new converts to prevention, having discovered that behaviour affects health, focus on the responsibility of the individual for illness prevention by eating and drinking in moderation, exercising properly, not smoking and the like. Surely, in the final analysis, it is the individual who carries out these actions. But what does it mean to hold the individual responsible for smoking when the government subsidizes tobacco farming, permits tax deductions for cigarette advertising and fails to use its taxing power as a disincentive to smoking? What does it mean to castigate the individual for poor eating habits when the public is inundated by advertisements for "empty-calorie" fast foods and is reinforced in present patterns of consumption by federal farm policy?' [51].

Using evidence

Scientific evidence has an incontestable role in public health in that it is essential to inform effective and appropriate actions, programmes and policies. However, there are serious challenges to acquiring good data [52], and when they do exist, they are not always independent and are seldom comparable, and merely having a set of data does not guarantee action on the part of decision makers. This makes it all the more difficult for the public health community to communicate risk clearly.

Understanding where data come from, and striving to base actions and initiatives on scientifically independent data, will be essential for public health practitioners. There is already substantial evidence from the literature on the health impact of tobacco that articles produced by the tobacco industry or by scientists supported by the tobacco industry are less objective. This is equally true in other areas such as food and nutrition. For example, Vartanian et al. carried out a systematic review of the effects of soft drink consumption on nutrition and health. They analysed the effect size as reported by industry-funded versus non-industry-funded studies on soft drinks and health and found that the average overall effect size for industry-funded studies was significantly smaller than the average effect size for non-industry-funded studies. When examining studies on the effects of soft drink consumption on energy intake, effect sizes were moderate for non-industry-funded studies and essentially non-existent for industry-funded studies [53]. It is the responsibility of the public health community to critically consider where the evidence comes from.

Even with the provision of robust independent data, action does not always follow evidence. Stone et al. propose several explanations as to why this might be [54]. There can be an inadequate supply of policy relevant research, a lack of access to research for both researchers and policy makers; poor policy comprehension by researchers concerning both the policy process and how research might be relevant to this process; ineffective communication by researchers of their work; a societal disconnection of both researchers and decision makers from those whom the research is about or intended for, to the extent that effective implementation is undermined; ignorance by policy makers about the existence of policy relevant research, or incapacity of overstretched bureaucrats to absorb research; poor governmental capacity to recognise and absorb research; power relations generating concerns about the contested validity of knowledge(s), issues of censorship and control and the question of ideology [54].

Policy-making is not a rational process, but rather messy and highly political; rarely is there a direct causal chain between the production of scientific evidence (or even the acknowledgement that there is a problem) and the development and implementation of relevant policies. As public health practitioners we need to understand the dynamic process and players in much greater depth.

Implications for public health practitioners

What are the specific actions that public health practitioners should initiate or continue to develop, in light of the current application of and debates within public health? Gray et al. [36] suggest that if there are still challenges in public health, and indeed where public health indices are worsening, this is due to an over-reliance on education and personal choice, and 'a failure to consider, or implement, other pivotal public health strategies such as regulation and fiscal intervention'. What are some of the ways forward for public health practitioners?

Be public health advocates

In light of some of the issues raised here, namely, that even solid evidence of a public health risk may not elicit adequate response from decision makers, and that some of the evidence generated may be coloured by vested interests, there is an important case to be made for public health advocacy [24]. As argued in a recent paper on public health advocacy [55], most fields of public health have objectives that can be strongly opposed by governments, industry, community and various interest groups, and even from within the public health field itself and so developing public health advocacy skills is crucial.

The disclosure of public health risks may cause some to lose significantly, either financially or in terms of social considerations [56]. Whose role is it to sound the alarm about the discovery or presumption of risk and to act upon it? This is exemplified in Henrik Ibsen's 1882 play 'An Enemy of the People' wherein the local doctor suggests that the town's lucrative spa be closed down because the surrounding waters are contaminated from nearby tanneries ('That source is poisoned [...] The whole of the town's prosperity is rooted in a lie!') and is met by angry opposition by local authorities: 'The matter in this instance is by no means a purely scientific one; it is a combination of technical and economic factors. [...] Any man who can cast such aspersions against his own birthplace is nothing but a public enemy' [57]. Practitioners and decision makers face a messy problem when confronting risk where the problem itself is ill-defined (or there is disagreement about how it should be defined). Some have particular interests in the problem, though the problem is often characterised by scientific uncertainty as noted above, and existing processes for solving the problem have, up to that point, proven insufficient. Significantly, while the problem in question may touch on health effects, inevitably it also touches upon social, political and economic issues [56]. Chapman proposes ten key questions to ask oneself as part of strategic planning for public health advocacy [55]:

(1) What are your public health objectives with this issue?
(2) Can a 'win-win' outcome be first engineered with decision makers?
(3) Who do the key decision makers answer to, and how can these people be influenced?
(4) What are the strengths and weaknesses of your and your opposition's position?
(5) What are your media advocacy objectives?
(6) How will you frame what is at issue here?
(7) What symbols or word pictures can be brought into this frame?
(8) What sound bites can be used to convey 6 and 7?
(9) Can the issue be personalised?
(10) How can large numbers of people be quickly organised to express their concerns?

Communicate public health risks effectively and to all stakeholders

A key element of public health advocacy is communication: in order to improve disease risk understanding across the board, one must address the many 'publics' in the real world [58]. Risk communication should keep in mind the particular positions of interested parties and be communicated without being prescriptive but by explaining the risks according to the priorities of each type of stakeholder. An important but often ignored fact is that there is no single 'public', particularly when it comes to communicating the health risks faced by individuals and communities at large: there are many different publics, not only in terms of sex, age and geography, but also in terms of individual risk susceptibility, exposure and risk literacy [58]. Those at greatest potential risk are often least likely to be well informed about the risks they face or be able to understand the complex, changing information about health hazards. On the other hand, those who actively seek out health information through the traditional mass media channels are a more literate audience and are often at lower risk because they are already taking good care of themselves and have access to healthier lifestyles and behaviours [58]. The European Food Information Council [59] suggests key pointers at getting the message across, including:

- **Know your target**: It is vital to be clear about their target audience. Is it the citizen, a stakeholder group, regulators, other trade bodies, or a combination of these actors?
- **Craft an appropriate message**: Know the nature of the risks to be communicated. Are they technical or naturally occurring, are they voluntary or involuntary, are they familiar or unfamiliar? The message can then be crafted accordingly. It is also important to pick the most appropriate communication tool for disseminating the message. In doing so, one must also carefully weigh the costs (public concern), and benefits (public reassurance) associated with each communication method.
- **Do not amplify risks or events**: By amplifying risks that are by their nature perceived as attenuated (most food risks fall in this category), a communication strategy is bound to fail; the audience will eventually see through any amplification and discard the message. Unnecessarily amplifying risks will be viewed as scare mongering and lead to public distrust in the source of the information.
- **Do not involve too many authorities**: Having two many groups involved increases the chance of having conflicting messages. This can lead to inflexibility, leaks and miscommunication, all contributing to public misunderstanding.
- **Proactive communication is best**: Proactive and transparent communication increases public trust and retroactive risk communication decreases it. On the other hand, communicating uncertainties when it is not necessary increases public confusion.

Source: Adapted from The European Food Information Council [59].

The current obesity epidemic exemplifies the challenge of effectively communicating the risk of not acting to prevent this disease. The literature and data have established obesity as a major public health issue, and one that is escalating in most countries of the world. They demonstrate how its origins extend beyond individual behaviour to encompass the 'obesogenic' environments that increasingly characterise modern societies. Britain is no exception; indeed, government figures suggest that two-thirds of adults and a third of children are either overweight or obese. These figures could rise to almost nine in ten adults and two-thirds of children by 2050, putting them at serious risk of heart disease, diabetes and cancer [60, 61]. However, in Britain as in other countries, information on the health impact of obesity has not in itself been sufficient to adequately move government to action, often because there are other, more urgent and more visible priorities on the agenda. Here, the cost argument may carry more weight with policy makers [62]: it is estimated that the pressure obesity and its associated illnesses and conditions put on families, the NHS and society more broadly with overall costs to society forecast to reach £ 50 billion per year by 2050 on current trends [63]. Preventing obesity leads to cost saving. An American study showed that a sustained 10% weight loss among obese people would translate into a lifetime saving of US $2200 to 5300 per person (1999 prices) depending on age, gender and starting body mass index, and an increase in life expectancy of 2-7 months. The study also found that lifetime incidence of coronary heart disease could be reduced from 12 to 1 case per 1000, and the incidence of stroke from 38 to 13 cases per 1000 [64].

Information is not enough

Merely providing information to consumers, patients and, as discussed above, government will not be enough to bring about changes in behaviour conducive to disease prevention and health promotion. Preventing disease risk is certainly not only a question of health education: effective action should engage with areas such as education, information, culture, trade, transport, distribution, industry and social services [65].

The tendency to understand the contexts within which populations live and work by involving different sectors and fields illustrates the fact that the scope and purpose of public health are still very political. As in the nineteenth century when public health actors and approaches were being formalised, there continues to be difficult debates because public health touches on areas with high stakes for different stakeholders at the local, national and international levels, such as tobacco, food and climate change. These three examples on their own comprise a series of important determinants of health (such as diet and nutrition, food-borne pathogens, the use of tobacco products, the impact of environmental deterioration on water and food sources and so forth) and their role in health (or lack thereof) of populations is for the most part grounded in robust scientific bases. However, they are particularly political subjects in part because the economic stakes are extremely high. Thus, simply imparting knowledge about these public health risks does not necessarily translate into action (arguably more often not). For example, narrow nutritional education has, on the whole, failed to change diet since it has focused traditionally on reducing risky behaviour through improving knowledge of individuals. Reviews of nutrition education interventions (see Box 1.1, for an example) find that while a focus on individual behavioural change may be effective in the short term, the factors influencing long-term changes are environmental, i.e. broad-based involvement of the school and the community [66, 74, 75].

Box 1.1   Factors of success in most effective interventions for fruit and vegetable consumption

A systematic review of the evidence of interventions to promote children's fruit and vegetable consumption found that the evidence is strongest in favour of multifaceted interventions [66].

A closer look at the three most effective reviewed studies [67–69] suggests that the more students are exposed to fruit and vegetables, the more the consumption patterns improve. Fruit and vegetable intake increases were highest with the most intensive exposure such as independent work in classrooms, canteens and with families, community youth organisation activities, point-of-purchase education and promotion in produce markets, public service announcements on local television stations, fruit and vegetable promotion competitions sponsored by the local fruit and vegetable industry, and providing links with local organisations in the community which offered low-cost nutrition and physical activity programmes for the parents.

Lessons learned from other areas of public health point to the importance of creating an enabling environment within which public health can be promoted [70]. It is important that an enabling environment for fruit and vegetable consumption by children be generated. This might include a range of macro-level interventions such as increasing access to fruit and vegetables through targeted government subsidies of production; agricultural policies that support healthy diets [71]; adequate funding and policies for schools to provide adequate school food services including local fresh fruit and vegetables [72], reduced access to junk food in schools to make the 'healthier choice' easier for children [73], and consistent practice (at least in the school) of nutrition education lessons.

Source: Adapted from Knai et al. [66].

Facilitating the participation of all stakeholders

Actors in public health include a series of stakeholders at the local, regional, national and international level. International organisations and agencies such as the European Commission and United Nations have a crucial role in raising public health issues on the political agenda. They can help coordinate, share good practice and monitor progress in countries and support national-level actions to reduce the ill health. Government ministries and agencies have a primary steering and stewardship role where they can build on existing structures and processes that address all aspects of public health, e.g. diet, nutrition and physical activity [76]. This stewardship role may be interpreted in many ways but the primary responsibility of governments for safeguarding public health is fundamental. The health sector often relies on conventional approaches involving health promotion programmes that have been found to achieve little success unless supported by regulation; it should rather call attention to the importance of public health as a key compound in overall strategic planning.

The academic and research institutions, from schools to universities and research centres, have a central role in knowledge generation and dissemination. They have a responsibility to produce independent research and inform evidence-based policy by working with other sectors, stakeholders and national/international health authorities such as the WHO.

Non-governmental organisations are key players particularly in monitoring the activities of organisations and institutions involved in public health activities and research. They can also help to ensure governments provide support for healthy lifestyles, and the food industry to provide more healthy products and services [76]. These organisations tend to still be traditionally 'low-influence' stakeholder groups, along with other civil society organisations, teachers and parents; they will need to develop their skills to ensure that they can contribute constructive and participatory responses to risk communication processes. If all stakeholders are to participate constructively, decision-making processes in public health need to better accommodate and formalise interactions with these groups [77]. How can this be done? Parents, teachers and school administrations can be unexpectedly influential at raising awareness and bringing about change, and this process should as far as possible be documented and analysed. Initiatives to support empowerment – enabling people to mobilise social forces and create conditions that are conducive to health living – are essential in making all voices heard and taken into account [65].

Summary

This chapter traces some of the various incarnations of public health since its inception as a field of study and practice, and highlights important milestones in our understanding of contemporary public health. The political commitments that have been taken during this time underscore the growing recognition that disease aetiology is more often than not complex and therefore warrants a multifaceted, comprehensive approach, with a focus on behaviour change and supportive environments and policies. The challenges, discussed in this chapter, are by no means exhaustive, but on their own they point to an increasing imperative for public health practitioners and governments to use the existing independent evidence and to act. This can be facilitated by building effective coalitions across relevant sectors and getting public support for appropriate, effective action in the promotion of healthy environments [36]. This is not an easy task, and as history reminds us, requires courage of conviction and political backing: 'from the early days of sanitary reform and slum clearance, there has always been opposition to public health action in one form or another. We need to recognise that the new public health challenges may bring us into conflict with different groups, which will include those with powerful vested interests. Building a robust consensus from across the political spectrum to support public health action where needed will be a key skill for the public health advocates of tomorrow' [36].

References

1 Jones L. *The Social Context of Health and Health Work*. Basingstoke: Macmillan, 1994.

2 World Health Organization. WHO definition of health. Preamble to the Constitution of the World Health Organization as adopted by the International Health Conference, New York, 19-22 June 1946; signed on 22 July 1946 by the representatives of 61 States (Official Records of the World Health Organization, no. 2, p. 100) and entered into force on 7 April 1948. Geneva: World Health Organization, 1946. Accessed August 2008 on http://www.who.int/about/definition/en/print.html.

3 Fox D. Politics as a tool of public and occupational health practice. In: Nelson M, ed. *Occupational Health and Public Health: Lessons from the Past - Challenges for the Future*, Nr 2006:10 (available at http://wwwmedicineguse/digitalAssets/824/824187_ah2006_10pdf). Stockholm: National Institute for Working Life, 2006.

4 Nelson M. *Occupational Health and Public Health: Lessons from the Past - Challenges for the Future*, Nr 2006:10 (available at http://www.medicine.gu.se/digitalAssets/824/824187_ah2006_10.pdf). Stockholm: National Institute for Working Life, 2006.

5 Viseltear A. CEA Winslow and the early years of public health at Yale, 1915-1925. *Yale Journal of Biological Medicine* 1982; **55**: 137-51.

6 Stirling A, Gee D. Science, precaution, and practice. *Public Health Reports* 2002; **117**(6): 521-33.

7 Beaglehole R, Bonita R. Public health at the crossroads: which way forward? *Lancet* 1998; **351**: 590-92.

8 Berridge V. History in the public health tool kit. *Journal of Epidemiology and Community Health* 2001; **55**: 611-12.

9 Wood F. The prophet in public health. *Public Health* 1928; **42**: 198-202.

10 Grieco A, Bock-Berti G, Fano D. Occupational health and public health: analogies and discrepancies. In: Nelson M, ed. *Occupational Health and Public Health: Lessons from the Past - Challenges for the Future*, Nr 2006:10 (available at http://wwwmedicineguse/digitalAssets/824/824187_ah2006_10pdf). Stockholm: National Institute for Working Life, 2006.

11 Beaglehole R, Bonita R. *Public Health at the Crossroads: Achievements and Prospects*, 2nd edn. Cambridge: Cambridge University Press, 2004.

12 Rosen G. *A History of Public Health*. Baltimore: The Johns Hopkins University Press, 1993.

13 Berridge V, Loughlin K. Public health history. *Journal of Epidemiology and Community Health* 2003; **57**: 164–5.

14 de Tocqueville A, Mayer J. *Journeys to England and Ireland*. London: Faber & Faber, 1958.

15 Morley I. City chaos, contagion, Chadwick, and social justice. *Yale Journal of Biological Medicine* 2007; **80**(2): 61–72.

16 Hamlin C. State medicine in Great Britain. In: Porter D, ed. *The History of Public Health and the Modern State*. Amsterdam: Editions Rodopi BV, 1994.

17 Chadwick E. *Report from the Poor Law Commissioners of an Enquiry into the Sanitary Conditions of the Labouring Population of Great Britain*. London, 1842. Excerpts accessed August 2008 on http://www.victorianweb.org/history/chadwick2.html.

18 Golub E. *The Limits of Medicine: How Science Shapes Our Hope for the Cure*. Chicago: University of Chicago Press, 1997.

19 Fee E, Porter D. Public health, preventive medicine and professionalization: England and America in the nineteenth century. In: Wear A, ed. *Medicine in Society*. Cambridge: Cambridge University Press, 1992.

20 Awofeso N. What's new about the "New Public Health"? *American Journal of Public Health* 2004; **94**(5): 705–9.

21 Rose G. *The Strategy of Preventive Medicine*. New York: Oxford University Press, 1993.

22 Marmot M, Wilkinson R. *Social Determinants of Health*. Oxford: Oxford University Press, 1999.

23 Cosgrove J. The McKeown thesis: a historical controversy and its enduring influence. *American Journal of Public Health* 2002; **92**(5): 725–9.

24 Pomerleau J, McKee M. *Issues in Public Health*. Maindehead: Open University Press, 2005.

25 World Health Organization. *Strategies for Health for All by the Year 2000* (available at http://www.wpro.who.int/rcm/en/archives/rc32/wpr_rc32_r05.htm). Geneva: World Health Organization, 1981.

26 World Health Organization. *From Alma-Ata to the Year 2000: Reflections at the Midpoint*. Geneva: World Health Organization, 1988.

27 World Health Organization. Ottawa Charter for Health Promotion. First International Conference on Health Promotion (Document WHO/HPR/HEP/ 95.1). Ottawa, 21 November 1986. Accessed September 2008 on http://www.who.int/hpr/NPH/docs/ottawa_charter_hp.pdf.

28 Stokols D. Establishing and maintaining healthy environments: toward a social ecology of health promotion. *American Psychologist* 1992; **47**: 6–22.

29 Sallis J, Owen N. Ecological models of health behavior. In: Glanz K, Rimer B, Lewis F, eds. *Health Behavior and Health Education: Theory, Research, and Practice*, 3rd edn, San Francisco: Jossey-Bass, 2002.

30 McLeroy K, Bibeau D, Steckler A, Glanz K. An ecological perspective on health promotion programs. *Health Education Quarterly* 1988; **15**: 351–77.

31 Sallis J, Cervero R, Ascher W, Henderson K, Kraft M, Kerr J. An ecological approach to creating active living communities. *Annual Review of Public Health* 2005; **27**: 297–322.

32 World Health Organization. *Diet, Nutrition and the Prevention of Chronic Diseases*. Report of a Joint WHO/FAO Expert Consultation. WHO Technical Report Series, No. 916. Geneva: World Health Organization, 2003.

33 World Health Organization. *Global Strategy on Diet, Physical Activity and Health*. Report by the Secretariat. 57th World Health Assembly (A57/9). Geneva: World Health Organization, 2004.

34 Association of Schools of Public Health. *This Is Public Health Toolkit*, 2008. Accessed August 2008 on http://www.thisispublichealth.org/toolkit/.

35 Centers for Disease Control and Prevention. Ten great public health achievements – United States, 1900–1999. *MMWR* 1999; **48**(12): 241–3. Accessed August 2008 on http://www.cdc.gov/mmwr/preview/mmwrhtml/00056796.htm.

36 Gray S, Pilkington P, Pencheon D, Jewell T. Public health in the UK: success or failure? *Journal of the Royal Society of Medicine* 2006; **99**: 107–11.

37 Office for National Statistics. *Life Expectancy*. Newport: Office for National Statistics, 2004. Accessed September 2008 on http://www.statistics.gov.uk/cci/nugget.asp?id=881.

38 Wanless D. *Securing Good Health for the Whole Population*. London: HM Treasury, 2004.

39 Parsons W. *Public Policy: An Introduction to the Theory and Practice of Policy*. Cheltenham, UK: Edward Elgar, 1995.

40 Mill J. *On Liberty*. New York: P.F. Collier & Son, 1860.

41 Hayek F. *The Road to Serfdom*. London: Routledge, 1944.

42 Rawls J. *A Theory of Justice*. Cambridge, MA: Harvard University Press, 1971.

43 Nozick R. *Anarchy, State and Utopia*. New York: Basic Books, 1974.

44 Booth S, Sallis J, Ritenbaugh C, Hill J, Birch L, Frank L et al. Environmental and societal factors affect food choice and physical activity: rationale, influences, and leverage points. *Nutrition Reviews* 2001; **3**: 21–39.

45 Egger G, Swinburn B. An 'ecological' approach to the obesity pandemic. *BMJ* 1997; **315**: 477–80.

46 French S, Story M, Jeffery R. Environmental influences on eating and physical activity. *Annual Review of Public Health* 2001; **22**: 309–25.

47 Tesh S. *Hidden Argument: Political Ideology and Disease Prevention Policy*. New Brunswick and London: Rutgers University Press, 1988.

48 Whitehead D, Russell G. How effective are health education programmes – resistance, reactance, rationality and risk? Recommendations for effective practice. *International Journal of Nursing Studies* 2004; **41**(2): 163–72.

49 Dowler E. Inequalities in diet and physical activity in Europe. *Public Health Nutrition* 2001; **4**(2B): 701–9.

50 McKee M, Raine R. Choosing health? First choose your philosophy. *Lancet* 2005; **365**: 369–71.

51 Eisenberg L. The perils of prevention: a cautionary note. *New England Journal of Medicine* 1977; **297**: 1231.

52 Pomerleau J, Knai C, Nolte E. The burden of chronic disease in Europe. In: Nolte E, McKee M, eds. *Caring for People with Chronic Conditions: A Health System Perspective*. Maidenhead: Open University Press, 2008.

53 Vartanian L, Schwartz M, Brownell K. Effects of soft drink consumption on nutrition and health: a systematic review and meta-analysis. *American Journal of Public Health* 2007; **97**(4): 667–75.

54 Stone D, Maxwell S, Keating M. *Bridging Research and Policy*. An international workshop funded by the UK Department for International Development. Warwick: Warwick University, 2001.

55 Chapman S. Advocacy for public health: a primer. *Journal of Epidemiology Community Health* 2004; **58**: 361–5.

56 Leviton C, Needleman C, Shapiro M. *Confronting Public Health Risks: A Decision Maker's Guide*. London: Sage, 1998.

57 Ibsen H. *An Enemy of the People*. Oxford: Oxford University Press, 1882.

58 Russell C. Implications for improving risk communication through various channels: a discussion. *National Cancer Institute Monograph* 1999; **25**: 177–8.

59 The European Food Information Council. *An Introduction to Food Risk Communication*. Accessed January 2007 on http://www.eufic.org/article/fr/Securite-
alimentaire-qualite-aliments/risk-communication/expid/review-food-risk-
communication/; EUFIC REVIEW(06), 2006.

60 Department of Health. *Healthy Weight, Health Lives: A Cross-Government
Strategy for England*. Accessed October 2008 on http://www.dh.gov.uk/en/
Publicationsandstatistics/Publications/PublicationsPolicyAndGuidance/
DH_082378; 2008.

61 NHS Information Centre. *Health Survey for England 2005 Latest Trends*.
London: NHS Information Centre, 2006.

62 Lang T, Rayner G. Overcoming policy cacophony on obesity: an ecological public
health framework for policymakers. *Obesity Reviews* 2007; **8**(Suppl 1): 165–81.

63 Foresight. *Tackling Obesities: Future Choices – Project Report*. London: Government Office for Science, 2007.

64 Oster G, Thompson D, Edelsberg J, Bird A, Colditz G. Lifetime health and economic benefits of weight loss among obese persons. *American Journal of Public
Health* 1999; **89**: 1536–42.

65 Vaandrager H, Koelen M. Consumer involvement in nutritional issues: the role
of information. *American Journal of Clinical Nutrition* 1997; **65**(Suppl): 1980S–
84S.

66 Knai C, Pomerleau J, Lock K, McKee M. Getting children to eat more fruit and
vegetables: a systematic review. *Preventive Medicine* 2006; **42**(2): 85–95.

67 Reynolds K, Franklin F, Binkley D, Raczynski J, Harrington K, Kirk K et al.
Increasing the fruit and vegetable consumption of fourth-graders: results from
the high 5 project. *American Journal of Preventive Medicine* 2000; **30**: 309–19.

68 Foerster S, Gregson J, Beall D, Hudes M, Magnuson H, Livingstone S et al. The
California children's 5 a day-power play! campaign: evaluation of large scale
social marketing initiative. *Family and Community Health* 1998; **21**: 46–64.

69 Gortmaker S, Cheung L, Peterson K, Chomitz G, Cradle J, Dart H et al. Impact
of a school-based interdisciplinary intervention on diet and physical activity
among urban primary school children: eat well and keep moving. *Archives of
Pediatrics and Adolescent Medicine* 1999; **153**(9): 975–83.

70 Swinburn B, Caterson I, Seidell J, James W. Diet, nutrition and the prevention of
excess weight gain and obesity. *Public Health Nutrition* 2004; **7**(Special Issue
1): 123–46.

71 Schafer-Elinder L. Public health aspects of the EU common agricultural policy.
In: *Developments and Recommendations for Change in Four Sectors: Fruit and
Vegetables, Dairy, Wine and Tobacco*. Stockholm: National Institute of Public
Health, 2003.

72 NHS. *The National School Fruit Scheme*. London: Department of Health, 2002.

73 James J, Thomas P, Cavan D, Kerr D. Preventing childhood obesity by reducing
consumption of carbonated drinks: cluster randomised controlled trial. *BMJ*
2004; **328**(7450): 1237.

74 Contento I. The effectiveness of nutrition education and implications for nutrition education policy, programs, and research: a review of research. *Journal
of Nutrition Education* 1995; **27**(6): 277–418.

75 Pomerleau J, Lock K, Knai C, McKee M. A systematic review of interventions
designed to increase adult fruit and vegetable intake. *Journal of Nutrition*
2005; **135**: 2486–95.

76 World Health Organization. Involving different stakeholders. In: Branca F, Niko-gosian H, Lobstein T, eds, *The Challenge of Obesity in the WHO European Region and the Strategies for Response.* Copenhagen: World Health Organization, Regional Office for Europe, 2007.

77 Robertson A, Tirado C, Lobstein T, Knai C, Jensen J, Ferro-Luzzi A et al. *Food and Health in Europe: A New Basis for Action.* WHO Regional Publications, European Series No 96. Copenhagen: WHO Regional Office for Europe, 2004. Accessed at http://www.euro.who.int/eprise/main/WHO/ Information-Sources/Publications/Catalogue/20040204_1.

Chapter 2
Public Health Nursing

Gill Coverdale

Learning objectives

After reading this chapter you will be able to:

- Define nursing and public health nursing
- Describe the role of the statutory bodies and the statutory and mandatory aspects of nursing registration
- Discuss the public health nursing role within health promotion
- Explore the four levels of prevention: primordial, primary, secondary and tertiary
- Comment on the challenges for public health nursing in the twenty-first century

Introduction

Chapter 1 looked at defining public health and argued that achieving public health is complex and the scope ill-defined; however, the large amount of effort that has gone into making public health a recognised field of practice has resulted in a range of practitioners contributing to this specialism. Elaine Haycock-Stuart says:

> An emerging conclusion is that for public health nursing to stand the test of time attention needs to be given to making explicit the knowledge that is informing the design of planned interventions and the framework for research and evaluation. It will be a missed opportunity if nursing seizes the opportunity to work extensively with a public health approach without simultaneously developing the theory behind its inception and evaluation. This is not a simple task, but a necessary one for nursing to be acknowledged for its contribution to meeting the public health agenda [1].

This chapter will look at the nursing contribution to public health and in particular those nurses registered on the third part of the Nursing and Midwifery

Council (NMC) register - specialist community public health nurses (SCPHNs). It will first analyse the definitions of nursing and public health nursing assessing the similarities and differences between the two. The role of the statutory bodies, the statutory and mandatory aspects of nursing registration and the relatively new public health part of the nursing register will be discussed. It will outline the role of the nursing professional bodies and the guidance and support they provide for their specific nursing disciplines. The public health nursing role within health promotion and the four levels of prevention: primordial, primary, secondary and tertiary will be explored and debated along with the challenges for public health nursing in the twenty-first century in the promotion of the health and well-being of the whole population.

The definition of nursing and public health nursing

Defining nursing

In 2003, the Royal College of Nursing (RCN) provided a comprehensive review to define 'nursing' using a national and international group of experts and wide consultation. It was felt that nursing required 'some specification for purposes such as the formulation of policy, the specification of services, and the development of educational curricula' [2, p. 1]. Interestingly, the United Kingdom Central Council (UKCC; the nursing regulation body at the time) suggested that a definition was not useful and would place restrictions on the profession. A definition was, however, agreed upon:

> The use of clinical judgement in the provision of care to enable people to improve, maintain, or recover health, to cope with health problems, and to achieve the best possible quality of life, whatever their disease or disability, until death. [2, p. 1]

Nursing encompasses a range of skills, attributes and competencies, and arguably requires the provision of empathy and sympathy towards the client/patient and their families. Nursing interventions are concerned with empowering people, and helping them to achieve, maintain or recover independence [2]. The RCN [2, p. 3] suggests that

> Nursing is an intellectual, physical, emotional and moral process which includes the identification of nursing needs; therapeutic interventions and personal care; information, education, advice and advocacy; and physical, emotional and spiritual support. In addition to direct patient care, nursing practice includes management, teaching, and policy and knowledge development.

Of course, nurses must and cannot avoid working in partnership - with patients, their relatives, other carers and even employers, as well as collaborating with others as members of a multidisciplinary/agency team. Leadership is a necessity and skills such as delegating, supervising the work of others and arguably prescribing are all skill sets the nurse requires and develops through their career pathway. However, nurses remain professionally accountable for their own decisions both on and off duty and issues such as confidentiality is second nature to a good nurse, which arguably is quite distinctive to the health care profession.

There are three parts to the NMC register: Nursing (Part 1), Midwifery (Part 2) and since 2004, Part 3 for SCPHNs, for those nurses with a predominantly public health role. Each part of the register has a designated title indicative of different qualifications and different kinds of education or training and a registrant is entitled to use the title corresponding to the part of the register in which they are registered [2].

In England there are three main disciplines on the public health part of the NMC register - health visitors (HVs), occupational health nurses (OHNs) and school nurses (SNs) - who each deliver services to a range of clients from primary and community care and in the school and work setting. The register is also open to sexual health nurses and those nurses with a predominantly public health role but who have not undertaken specific specialist programmes. This chapter will focus on the collective role of nurses registered on this part of the NMC register who will be collectively termed SCPHNs for ease of writing. Later chapters will explore the distinctive roles of health visiting, occupational health nursing and school nursing with the literature, research and policy directives for each discipline.

Defining public health nursing

The NMC states that the third part of the register

> ...recognises those nurses who work with populations and whose role is primarily public health focused - including the responsibility to work with both individuals and a population, which may mean taking decisions on behalf of a community or population without having direct contact with every individual in that community. [3, p. 4]

This provides a different emphasis to the role of the general nurse in that the SCPHN may not necessarily work with individuals but rather a community or population group who they will not meet all members of; when they do work with individuals these are often referred to as clients. These clients most likely *choose* to engage in professional help and advice as they are not a captive audience as in hospital or requiring care after illness or medical intervention. The difference is notable as the SCPHN may be viewed in a very different manner if help or advice has not been actively sought by the client.

The elements of public health nursing are:

- Planning health promoting and health protecting programmes
- Reducing risky behaviours and health inequalities
- Preventing disease

- Assessing and monitoring the health of communities and populations to identify those at risk and those with health problems
- Assessing health needs and identify priorities for action

The principles of public health nursing are centred on equity, collaboration and participation with others to strengthen community action [4]. As capacity for services in the acute sector becomes more constrained, the need for preventative action in the community is increased. Securing healthy lifestyle actions which provide short- and subsequent long-term benefits for people are vital. It is argued that the public health role of nurses needs strengthening so that every contact is an opportunity to promote health regardless of the setting [5]. An essence of care benchmark on promoting health [6] has been developed to ensure quality is being driven into service provision. SCPHNs provide care along the continuum of public health practice working with the individual through the differing population groups; working with children laying down the foundations of good health or supporting and managing the chronically sick; changing unhealthy lifestyles, improving knowledge or attitudes, personal empowerment, or influencing policy and community development [7].

SCPHNs need to be responsive to the needs of both individuals and population groups, working with communities and other agencies in order to meet need. In order to do this effectively, they have to lead community public health nursing practice within their communities. A community is defined by the NMC [3] as a group of people living or working in a geographically defined area or who have a characteristic, cause, need or experience in common. An empathic understanding that the behaviours of their population groups are influenced by social and environmental factors, cultural norms and economy, as well as policy and politics is vital as these factors deem to shape the choices their client groups make and the environments they live in [8].

The determinants of health are firmly rooted in the lives of the SCPHN's client groups and promoting and maintaining public health is about enabling and empowering these population groups to have influence over these health and social determinants. The World Health Organization (WHO) asserts that empowerment is a process through which people gain greater control over decisions and actions affecting their health. It may be a social, cultural, psychological or political process through which individuals and social groups are able to express their needs, present their concerns, devise strategies for involvement in decision making, and achieve political, social and cultural action to meet those needs [9].

The influence of policy

National government policy has recognised the public health contribution of all nurses, midwives and HVs [10–15] and advocates a range of policy to drive the agenda forward in improving public health services [16–19]. Nurses have a major role to play in promoting the health of their client groups and are seen as advocates, enabling and advising clients on their health and well-being [14, 15].

The Ottowa Charter [20] is a vital guide for health-promoting nursing practice, and as public health is everyone's business, the role of public health promotion is a major role for all nurses who need to ensure wherever they practice that they are in a position to adopt public health practices in their work. This is reflected in their roles and responsibilities of health education for restoration and promotion of health and prevention of disease; participation in preventive measures and programmes; and epidemiological surveys [21].

The SCPHN is required to be politically active with the ability to:

> ...contribute to the development of public policies in collaboration with community and government leaders. These policies are designed to solve identified local priorities and address national health problems. If nurses are to influence policy they need to understand the political and ideological interplay that influences and drives service provision.

Richman [22] proposes that there are three key perspectives changing the face of public health and therefore impacting on the provision and delivery of public health nursing services:

- The population groups as consumers are taking responsibility for their own health
- The power relationship between the consumer and the health professional has changed and the health professional is no longer solely responsible for providing expert advice and support
- Health care is not confined to large institutions such as the NHS

It is, therefore, not just about assuring that populations have access to appropriate and cost-effective care, which includes health promotion and disease prevention services and evaluation of the effectiveness of that care; it is also essential to address health and social inequalities such as general socioeconomic, cultural and environmental conditions, living and working conditions and social and community influences. This requires nurses to take into account individual lifestyle factors, age, sex and genetic influences. Enabling individuals and communities to take charge of their own health should be a key aim in all public health nursing, but this requires multi-agency collaborative working; it cannot be done solely by one agency. Partnerships also need to be encouraged with the individuals in a community to help shape the services provided to meet their needs. The call for health needs assessments carried out in partnership with client groups, as the way forward in helping to identify local needs, is prevalent in the literature [23-26].

Ideology of public health practice

In order for intersectoral partnerships to develop, communication and interpersonal skills are essential, as is an understanding of the ideology, structure and philosophy of public health practice within the differing professional roles, as well as an awareness of the constraints for delivering public health. There is much written on the ideologies of public health and a brief introduction would need to include three broad ideological perspectives offered by Baggott [27]:

- Collectivism/socialism
- Environmental/green ideology
- Individualism/libertarianism

Baggott [27] asserts that collectivists and socialists place great emphasis on the role of the state, voluntary societies and cooperative efforts and are cynical of the ability of the individual to produce their own solutions to complex social problems. They see the role of the state as integral to the amelioration of health-damaging behaviours of individuals. Equity in health is their key aim to achieve social justice; state intervention is therefore justified to reduce junk food, emissions, smoking in public places and alcohol consumption; and promotes everyone's health regardless of social class, income, gender, or ethnicity [27]. It could be argued that current health policy is leaning towards this 'nanny-state' approach with individual health promotion as well as community-based action.

Environmentalists, or those adopting a green perspective, oppose the destruction of society through economic growth and industrialisation, relying on individuals and groups to promote a sustainable environment [27]. They are proponents of social justice and the power of collectivism; however, they are wary of state power, believing it to be oppressive towards individuals and as damaging to the environment if it suits. A collective responsibility for improving health and making cities and towns more healthy places to live in is arguably necessary as individual interventions alone does not prevent 'some cities making you sick' [28].

Individualists and libertarians believe in negative liberty and that individuals have a right to pursue their own activities without interference from the state, providing others are not harmed [27]. They call for an increase in individual responsibility through informed choice. They argue that this can achieve 'healthism', which at its most powerful facilitates the domination of individuals away from the 'experts'.

This requirement to consider one's own ideological perspective as a practitioner can facilitate an understanding of how much one's own personal perspective actually influences the way care is delivered to the client groups. This also has an enormous impact when working with a group of professionals from different agencies, all with differing attitudes and values on top of individual ideological perspectives. This can be a challenge and is not always addressed when multi-agency work is being planned and implemented.

The role of the statutory bodies: the statutory and mandatory aspects of SCPHN registration

Most countries have a legal definition of the title 'nurse' and some also have a legal definition of 'nursing'. In the UK there is no legal definition of 'nursing', but 'registered nursing care' has been defined by the Health and Social Care Act 2001 [2] in such a way that it can be distinguished from 'social care' or 'personal care' for the purpose of defining responsibility for its provision and eligibility for funding. This legislative definition, however, does not relate in any way to professional definitions or to specifications of the nurse's scope of practice [2].

The NMC

The NMC was established under the Nursing and Midwifery Order 2001 [29] and came into being on 1 April 2002 as the successor to the United Kingdom Central Council for Nursing, Midwifery and Health Visitors (UKCC) and the four National Boards for Nurses, Midwives and Health Visitors for England, Northern Ireland, Scotland and Wales. One of the principal functions of the NMC is to establish and monitor standards of education and training and assess conduct and performance for nurses and midwives. This will ensure the maintenance of standards and importantly safeguard the health and well-being of persons using or needing the services of nurses and midwives on the register [29].

The NMC is responsible for regulating and assuring the public of safe, effective nursing and midwifery practice and has set standards for registration to provide the mechanism through which the NMC can exercise its main function of protecting the public [30]. The NMC maintain that whilst pre-registration education provides nurses with the knowledge, skills and attitudes to give safe and effective care, professional practice alone following registration is not enough to meet the additional needs of specialist practitioners. Standards have been set for both community specialist practice [31], which remains a recordable qualification, and specialist community public health nursing [3], which is a qualification, which requires registration as the NMC takes the view that this form of practice has distinct characteristics that require public protection [3]. Those who achieve the standards of proficiency are eligible to apply to enter the third part of the NMC register for SCPHNs. The context in which the standards are achieved defines the scope of professional practice within each practitioner's identified area of community public health nursing [3].

Standards of proficiency for specialist community public health nursing [3]

The programme preparing the SCPHN is guided by four main principles taken from the health visiting principles [32] which establish the philosophy and values underpinning the profession and are outlined in brief:

- **Preparation:** Ensuring nurses are fit to practice – developed through practice-centred learning, theory and practice integration and evidence-based practice and learning.

- **Service:** Ensuring nurses are fit for purpose developed through the management of community public health services which are provided on a needs basis, focused on social groups, whilst acknowledging the practitioner's need to extend the scope of practice through lifelong learning.
- **Recognition:** Ensuring nurses are fit for the award through the provision of high-quality academic programmes of no less than degree level in a practice-centred educational environment.
- **Responsibility**: Ensuring nurses are fit for professional standing through adherence to the NMC code of professional conduct, performance and ethics [30].

These principles provide the foundation for SCPHN programmes ensuring the standards of proficiency for entry to the register are achieved. Article 5(a) [2] of the Order [29] requires the NMC to:

> establish the standards of proficiency necessary to be admitted to the different parts of the register being the standards it considers necessary for safe and effective practice under that part of the register. [3, p. 9]

These standards of proficiency [3] (Table 2.1) underpin the ten key principles of public health practice in the context of specialist community public health nursing. They are grouped into four domains containing 23 standards which students must achieve proficiency, competence and confidence in:

- Search for health needs
- Stimulation of awareness of health needs
- Influence on policies affecting health
- Facilitation of health-enhancing activities

The role of professional bodies

There are numerous professional bodies supporting public health nurses in a field of nursing distinct from the other routes straddling medicine, education, the workplace and children's social services. These professional bodies provide support in various ways, some with union services and membership. All the groups work closely with key decision makers in the Department of Health, NHS trusts across the UK and other professional and political organisations.

The RCN

The RCN represents nurses from all disciplines of the profession and is their voice locally, nationally and internationally. Amongst its aims is to promote excellence in practice and shape health policies; influence and lobby governments and others to develop and implement policy that improves the quality

Table 2.1 Standards of proficiency for entry to the register.

Principle	Domain
	Search for health needs
Surveillance and assessment of the population's health and well-being	Collect and structure data and information on the health and well-being and related needs of a defined population
	Analyse, interpret and communicate data and information on the health and well-being and related needs of a defined population
	Develop and sustain relationships with groups and individuals with the aim of improving health and social well-being
	Identify individuals, families and groups who are at risk and in need of further support
	Undertake screening of individuals and populations and respond appropriately to findings
	Stimulation of awareness of health needs
Collaborative working for health and well-being Working with, and for, communities to improve health and well-being	Raise awareness about health and social well-being and related factors, services and resources
	Develop, sustain and evaluate collaborative work
	Communicate with individuals, groups and communities about promoting their health and well-being
	Raise awareness about the actions that groups and individuals can take to improve their health and social well-being
	Develop capacity and confidence of individuals and groups, including families and communities, to influence and use available services, information and skills, acting as advocate where appropriate
	Work with others to protect the public's health and well-being from specific risks
	Influence on policies affecting health on policies affecting health
Developing health programmes and services and reducing inequalities	Work with others to plan, implement and evaluate programmes and projects to improve health and well-being
	Identify and evaluate service provision and support networks for individuals, families and groups in the local area or setting
Policy and strategy development and implementation to improve health and well-being	Appraise policies and recommend changes to improve health and well-being
	Interpret and apply health and safety legislation and approved codes of practice with regard for the environment, well-being and protection of those who work with the wider community
	Contribute to policy development

(Continued)

Table 2.2 (*Continued*)

Principle	Domain
Research and development to improve health and well-being	Develop, implement, evaluate and improve practice on the basis of research, evidence and evaluation
	Facilitation of health-enhancing activities
Promoting and protecting the population's health and well-being	Work in partnership with others to prevent the occurrence of needs and risks related to health and well-being
	Work in partnership with others to protect the public's health and well-being from specific risks
	Prevent, identify and minimise risk of interpersonal abuse or violence, safeguarding children and other vulnerable people, initiating the management of cases involving actual or potential abuse or violence where needed
Developing quality and risk management within an evaluative culture	Prevent, identify and minimise risk of interpersonal abuse or violence, safeguarding children and other vulnerable people, initiating the management of cases involving actual or potential abuse or violence where needed
Strategic leadership for health and well-being	Apply leadership skills and manage projects to improve health and well-being
	Plan, deliver and evaluate programmes to improve the health and well-being of individuals and groups
Ethically managing self, people and resources to improve health and well-being	Manage teams, individuals and resources ethically and effectively

of patient care and health outcomes, and builds on the importance of nurses, health care assistants and nursing students. As well as this, they have an important role to play in supporting and protecting the value of nursing staff in all their diversity and educating nurses professionally and academically, building a resource of professional expertise and leadership. It is the largest nursing union. There are over 30 professional forums an RCN member can join, bringing like-minded professionals together to debate key issues. Interestingly, there is no forum specifically dedicated to public health nurses.

The Community Practitioners and Health Visitors Association

The Community Practitioners and Health Visitors Association (CPHVA) is the UK professional body that represents registered nurses and HVs who work in a primary or community health setting and recently suitably qualified nursery nurses have been able to join the CPHVA. It is part of the Unite trade union with two million members nationwide. Unite was formed by an amalgamation of Amicus and the Transport and General Workers' Union and is the third largest professional nursing union. Unite/CPHVA campaigns to protect the status of the community practitioner and the services they deliver. Unite/CPHVA influences policy decisions by the production of high-quality reports and consultation documents, as well as by the staging of conferences and seminars.

Professional forums

The three pathways also have professional forums. The United Kingdom Standing Conference (UKSC) is a body representing public health nursing in the UK, but was primarily developed to meet HV education and development needs. It provides a forum for discussion, exchange of information and news about meetings, conferences, seminars, workshops and other events on topics related to public health nursing education and practice and links to resources containing research and other information of interest from the four countries. A number of issues have recently been identified by UKSC for debate and research and at present these remain health visiting focused. These include:

- The focus of health visiting activity
- The goals for health visiting
- The core activities for health visiting
- The pre-requisites for effective practice
- Preparation for the role

The Association of Occupational Health Nurse Educators (AOHNEs) in the UK is an organisation for teachers of occupational health nursing at higher education institutions in UK. The organisation exists to promote best practice and education in occupational health nursing. It works closely with the NMC, the RCN and other professional and statutory bodies in order to ensure that education in occupational health reflects the needs of the workplace in a changing society. Through practice educators and mentors, AOHNE also collaborates with employers and their representatives in order to ensure the highest level of training, both in theory and practice.

The National Forum for School Health Educators (NFSHEs) is an organisation for teachers of school nursing in higher education institutions. Among the forum's aims are to inform and advise appropriate bodies at local, regional and national levels on issues relating to the education and training of school health practitioners in a bid to establish equity and parity of educational standards and to raise the profile of the work of school health practitioners.

Other associations are available for practitioners such as the School and Public Health Nurses Association (SAPHNA), which was officially launched on 1 January 2006, to provide a professional organisation that is dedicated to public health nurses' professional needs. It is dedicated to the promotion of excellence in practice, taking forward the public health agenda by working in partnerships for the benefit of children and young people and the communities where they live and learn. This is facilitated through the dissemination of a journal, conference/events, bulletins, website, research and other activities with key stakeholder groups.

Specialist occupational health bodies include the Association of Occupational Health Nurse Practitioners which has a marvellous website devoted to courses, events, related documents and developments in the field and a members-only section offering special offers and discounts. The Federation of Occupational Health Nurses in Europe is also a useful resource for the OHN.

The developing role of public health: prevention and health promotion

In the nineteenth century, public health work became more about improving social conditions and preventive medicine became focused on environmental health issues, understanding the effects of environment on health and of the link between poverty and health. In the early twentieth century, concern was placed on maternal and child health and community nursing services such as health visiting, district nursing and school nursing began to grow as health education and health inequalities became important. Around the same time, there was a focus on the health of workers and early inspections of health and safety was being addressed by at first doctors and then industrial nurses. The World War II became the final catalyst to push the country towards a welfare state. The evacuees pouring from London were in very poor health, infested and undernourished and it prompted a public outcry. War brought cohesion and even the wealthy had to accept the need to care for one's own countrymen. The 1942 Beveridge Report [33] on social services pleaded for the eradication of the five giants on the road to reconstruction – Want, Squalor, Idleness, Ignorance and Disease. This report amongst others recommended the creation of the NHS and the welfare state – a system of care that was comprehensive, inclusive and free at the point of delivery.

Public health medicine is traditionally associated with the prevention of disease through epidemiology and surveillance, what we perceive as a medical model of health. The independent inquiry into inequalities in health [34] took a social model of health and made 39 recommendations. Thirty-six of these ranged across the whole spectrum of government policy that influenced health inequalities. A cross-cutting review on health inequalities was then conducted by the Treasury with the participation of 18 government departments and agencies.

There are three domains in the modern faculty of public health work according to the Health Protection Agency:

- Health protection – protecting people from hazards, which damage their health: infectious diseases, chemicals and poisons, radiation, environmental health hazards, emergency response

- Health improvement - tackling inequalities, education, housing, employment, family/community issues, lifestyles, surveillance and monitoring of
  specific diseases and risk factors, screening
- Service improvement - clinical effectiveness, efficiency, service planning,
  audit and evaluation, clinical governance

The SCPHN role in health promotion

Prevention and health promotion remain key roles for nurses; prevention of
disease, disability or illness, and it is well recognised that they are in an ideal
position to deliver health promotion programmes both within hospital and
in the wider community, successfully contributing to the development of a
healthy population [11, 12, 35-37]. Enabling and empowering individuals and
groups is a key construct in the health-promoting role of nurses. Tones and
Green [38] suggest that health promotion emerged in response to meeting
the environmental and behavioural determinants of health 'making healthy
choices easy choices'. They offer a formula: Health Promotion = Healthy Public Policy × Health Education, which requires a symbiotic relationship between
education, social and political change. They assert that health promotion is
on the one hand the prevention and control of premature death and disease,
and on the other hand the promotion of well-being and control over health
through empowerment and enabling of individuals [38]. However, complex
psychosocial and socioeconomic factors, such as financial standing, education and motivation, can make it difficult for individuals to make healthy
choices. It is purported that telling people how we think they should live is
a moral and political process and educating people about their health should
be done through public forums, which highlight the inequalities in health and
the inequity in power distribution [39]. Arguably, people who can exercise
the greatest degree of autonomy will enjoy improved health [39, p. 302].
Laverack [40] also discusses the role power plays in health promotion and
public health and provides a useful guide on improving clients' power base
arguing that clients who have more power will gain more control over their
lives.

The NMC [3, p. 10] standards require the SCPHN to:

Develop and sustain relationships with groups and individuals with the aim of
improving health and social well-being; and develop capacity and confidence
of individuals and groups, including families and communities, to influence
and use available services, information and skills, acting as advocate where
appropriate.

The above skills and competence are vital if clients and communities are to
take on board health-promoting messages which will prevent illness, disease
or disability. Public health nursing should also operate at the 'pre-need' stage,
with public health nurses proactively addressing health need by identifying
self-declared, recognised and unrecognised health needs of individuals and

social groups. Particular attention needs to be paid to disadvantaged or vulnerable populations, health inequalities and other factors that contribute to health and well-being in the context of people's lives [3].

Prevention and the SCPHN

Preventative programmes in the last century in the UK have included improved sanitation, water supply and quality of food, housing and workplace conditions [41]. The pattern of health and illness has changed and historic infectious diseases such as cholera and smallpox are no longer a threat; however, chronic ill health and long-term conditions have replaced these concerns. Prevention of infectious diseases has been addressed via successful immunisation programmes in the UK; however, in other less developed countries diseases such as cholera, typhoid, measles, tuberculosis and malaria are still very much major killers. In the UK, we still live with the threat of tuberculosis especially as wide-scale immunisation has ceased. Of course, infectious disease is still with us from different types of infectious disease – MRSA, *Clostridiums difficile* and sexually transmitted diseases such as HIV/AIDS. Arguably, with increased globalisation and people travelling both for pleasure and for business and/or working abroad, there is an increasing risk of infectious diseases being brought to the UK population.

In addition to all these, at the top of the health care agenda are the chronic illnesses from our modern lifestyle, which are arguably more difficult to prevent:

- Obesity leading to circulatory disease and diabetes
- Smoking leading to lung cancer
- Increased drinking leading to liver cirrhosis
- Complex societal factors leading to mental health issues such as stress-related illnesses of anxiety and depression

Prevention of these modern life-threatening illnesses depends upon the action and motivations of the individual, although community interventions such as the 'smoking in public places ban' will help the fight against the effects of passive smoking. Beaglehole and Bonita [42] argue that with coronary heart disease becoming a leading cause of death in developed countries by 2020, the need for public health practice to maintain and strengthen the response to the modern non-communicable diseases of cancer, heart disease, stroke and diabetes requires a broad and sustained approach which takes into account the influence of socioeconomic factors.

There are four types of prevention that public health practitioners are involved in delivering – primordial, primary, secondary and tertiary. The first two relate to the prevention of disease and the second two in the promotion of quality of life. These are outlined below.

Primordial prevention

Primordial prevention is considered to be work that is carried out to prevent the development of disease at its earliest stages or early intervention work with those considered at increased risk in the first place. Its aim is to avoid the emergence and establishment of socioeconomic and cultural lifestyles that contribute to disease and includes the involvement of national and cross-cutting government policy [43]. A review was carried out to consider how having knowledge of the genetic causes of early cardiovascular disease can lead to directed screening and better treatment of high-risk individuals [44]. The study argued that while gene therapy would be the most 'primordial' approach to prevention of some diseases its practical application remains on the horizon and the use of epidemiology is integral to primordial prevention [44]. The collection of epidemiological data such as mortality and morbidity rates allows mapping of the incidence and spread and relates to known causes of disease, thus allowing priorities to be set which provides key information for public health practitioners to plan and implement primary prevention programmes [44]. They go on to argue that data must be collected, analysed and utilised in a regular and systematic way and can provide a prediction of the future disease burden and evaluate the success of disease prevention and health-promoting programmes. A good example of primordial prevention is the National Food in Schools Programme [45] implemented by the Department for Education and Skills which influences healthier food consumption in children and young people.

Primary prevention

This is aimed at limiting the incidence of disease by controlling specific causes and risk factors and is usually aimed at whole population groups or high-risk groups [43]. Good examples of primary prevention programmes are immunisations which provide immunity to diseases and prevent the onset of disease. The new HPV vaccine is a good example of such a vaccine which will prevent cervical cancer. Health promotion and advice programmes are also an example of primary prevention.

Secondary prevention

This aims to reduce the serious consequences of disease through early diagnosis and treatment [43]. These are measures that detect diseases early and commence strategies which will prevent its further progression. This is successful with diseases that have an early onset period that is not life-threatening such as screening programmes for cervical cancer where abnormal cells can be identified and effective action taken to prevent progression. Other good examples are screening programmes such as vision and hearing in workplaces and schools.

Tertiary prevention

This is aimed at reducing the progress or complications associated with the disease or illness by modifying behaviour and lifestyle and ensuring effective drug/nursing/medical intervention. This is an important aspect of the thera-peutic role of the nurse in reducing suffering and rehabilitating clients back to work or to adjusting to living a life with chronic disease. There will be more about this in Chapters 7 and 8.

The challenges for public health nursing

Delivering the public health agenda requires a workforce that is skilled and equipped to address the complex issues affecting the health of the public. The chief medical officer promotes three tiers in the public health workforce [46]:

- The general public health workforce – any one in the business of promoting health for instance nurses, doctors, social workers, teachers, police and others
- Public health practitioners – those spending a major part of their time in public health practice such as SCPHNs, other public health nurses and public health practitioners
- Public health specialists – specialist medical officers, specialist registrars and those senior strategists in public health

Skills, knowledge and competencies

SCPHNs practice in this complex and multi-layered environment and as nurses they form one of the largest groups of professionals promoting public health. It is, therefore, particularly important that they have skills and competencies in this field [47, 48]. Measurement of skills is arguably complex, yet there are tools which can assess and audit these skills. Elliston and Wilkinson produced and piloted a tool, which all practitioners could use to assess skills and identify training needs [47]. Their audit highlighted the need for management and leadership skills, resource issues, education, training and development. The paper called for mentorship, greater connectivity between regional and local practice, multi-professional education and a fresh look at the level of support for public health nurses.

A small unpublished qualitative research project carried out in 2006 [49] used a focus group approach to explore the knowledge, understanding and views of registered SCPHNs who are all active practice teachers for students undertaking the degree programme leading to the qualification. Participants were taken from health visiting, occupational health nursing and school nurs-ing and were asked to explore three key areas:

- Their public health role
- What the influences on that role are
- What they felt the solutions were to enhance this aspect of their role

The results of the research showed that the participants were knowledge-able about their role as public health nurses, but were influenced by lack of resources, poor understanding from others of their role and tensions with managers and the wider team as to the importance of their public health role. They offered solutions including role clarity for the skill mix team, a clear and joint vision for practice, and debated the idea of one member of the team taking on a specific public health nurse role. However, as it is unpublished and not yet peer reviewed its results should be interpreted with caution.

Lack of educational preparation is a theme throughout the literature and Danielson et al. [21] acknowledged this in their work and have developed a new educational framework for developing public health nurses with the key constructs being to develop skills in health needs assessment, epidemiology, health promotion, empowerment, advocacy, policy development, collaboration and evaluation. These are all reflected in the standards set by the NMC for SCPHNs and supported unanimously by other literature [3, 16, 21, 49–56] suggesting nurses working in public health require the theoretical skills and practical knowledge to work in community partnerships and interdisciplinary teams; to facilitate change; conduct population and community health needs assessments; develop and improve health promotion and disease prevention programmes; and advocate politically to help communities fulfil their health potential.

Plews et al.'s [54] research with nurses, lead nurses and managers revealed a limited knowledge and skills in public health promotion; that the interpretation of what public health is, was variable; the lack of collaboration between and within organisations and disciplines and community trusts was variable; and they were a long way off audit and evaluation of public health work. A common theme through the literature revealed nurses' feelings of being undervalued and underutilised, and Hemstrom (cited in Ref. [50]) suggests that this may be due to under publishing of successful work and to the obscurity of public health work in a highly technical biomedicalised health care system. There is also a common view that it is women's work, third rate and low graded [51, 55]. It is argued that the difficulties faced by community and public health nurses are due to the culture and paradigm of public health – the prevention of illness and promotion of health within a deep sociopolitical dimension, in competition with a prevailing illness model [57]. Also, in addition, the medical focus of general practitioners being on infection control and epidemiology, all of which serve to make public health more difficult to operationalise [54].

The population focus

What is common to all the literature is an acceptance that public health nursing in the new public health arena is population-based and prevention-focused with a number of challenges represented by the population it serves. Yet, Grumbach et al.'s [52] research found that the population focus is not reflected in public health nurses practice activities, management priorities or education preparation and in fact there was little systematic evidence of what constituted public health nursing practice at all. Holistic health and well-being must be achieved by the majority in the pursuit and promotion of a healthy population and this requires a shift in the acknowledgment that preventative medicine alone is not sufficient. An increased awareness of the need for social and community care, which takes into account the social and financial determinants and inequities of communities, is required. This was explored and highlighted by Black in 1980 [58] and Acheson in 1989 [59] and 1998 [34], with policy and politics playing a major role in the promotion of health. Recent government documentation exploring each of the disciplines separately will be addressed in more detail in later chapters but there are several key documents which explore the delivery of HV, OH and SN services in the twenty-first century [60, 62]. The *Tackling Health Inequalities: 2007 Status Report on the Programme for Action* [63] pursues this paradigm as health and social inequalities continue to exist well into the twenty-first century and 'remain stubborn, persistent and difficult to change' (p. 3) and provides up-to-date information on a range of key indicators as can be seen in the brief examples given in Box 2.1. These have been chosen as these represent key health promotion work for public health nurses.

Box 2.1 **Summary of progress against national indicators**

The big killers - Improvements in cancer and circulatory disease death rates since 1995–1997 (including for the most disadvantaged areas), with a narrowing of inequalities in absolute terms for both. No significant change in relative terms for cancer, but there has been a widening in inequalities in relative terms for circulatory diseases.

Teenage pregnancy - 13.3% drop in the rate of under-18 conceptions between 1998 and 2006 (with the average rate for the most disadvantaged areas also falling), with a slight narrowing of inequalities in absolute terms but no significant narrowing in relative terms.

Road accident casualties - Improvements in child road accident casualty rates since 1998 (including for the most disadvantaged areas). There has been a narrowing of inequalities in absolute terms, but no significant change in relative terms.

Smoking - Since 1998, smoking prevalence among all adults has fallen (including among manual groups), but there has been no significant change in inequalities for manual groups compared to non-manual groups or all adults in absolute terms, with some signs of a widening in relative terms.

Between 2000 and 2005, the overall prevalence of smoking throughout pregnancy decreased slightly, including a large fall in prevalence among women in the 'never worked' category but a slight increase among routine and manual groups. There were some signs of a widening of inequalities for routine and manual groups.

Fruit and vegetable consumption - Between 2001 and 2006, consumption of five or more portions of fruit and vegetables per day increased (including for households with the lowest incomes), but there was no significant change in inequalities between households with the lowest incomes and households with the highest incomes or the average for all households.

Clinical work versus public health work

The difficulties faced by public health nurses are increased by the tension in delivering the clinical role and the public health role, which was discussed by all my focus group participants and is also seen in Elliston and Wilkinson's [47] study which identified an emerging conflict of role - clinical caseload versus implementation and participation in public health practice. DeBell and Tomkins [64] argue that the literature and research from within public health nursing practice suggests that the terms public health, health promotion and health education are often used interchangeably. Although many nurses do carry out health-promoting initiatives, these are often aimed at the individual rather than the population, or they may be aimed at structural or organisational change. But they argue that most work is aimed at personal decision making and ensuring individuals have access to accurate information. Health surveillance is a key public health nursing role and is prevalent within the three key disciplines, for some groups it may require the skill of a specialist nurse whilst in other areas it is argued by practitioners as a task which can be taken on within the skill mix team and prevents more proactive work being carried out.

There have been crucial policy drivers in reorienting the NHS and Primary Care Trusts (PCTs) towards health promotion [10-16, 46] with nurses being integral to shifting the focus of public health from a medical/clinical perspective, to a community level, which takes into account the broader social health of the public and provides a framework to consider the social and political agenda. However, even with £1b financial input [65] to support new public health nursing roles, the 'non ring fencing' of this money meant it was diverted and has resulted in PCTs lacking the capacity to undertake public health work despite it being high on the policy agenda [65]. For OH delivery outside of the NHS this may not be seen as a major challenge but working outside of the NHS brings with it many other constraints which have been discussed and highlighted in Dame Carol Black's recent review of the health of Britain's working population [61].

Improving the role – what are the solutions?

The literature [21, 49-55] offers various solutions for improving the public health contribution of nurses:

- Marketing of skills and increased publication and research output
- Strategic health authorities and PCTs taking a critical appraisal of organisational and financial constraints
- Commissioners needing to define the public health role of its service providers
- Education programmes needing to educate for population health management, publication, research and marketing of the role and the skills to work in partnership and collaboration
- Managers needing to be clear on the future of public health nursing and ensure capacity, restructuring and reprioritisation

The skills for health agency and the NMC have addressed the need for competence through the setting of standards of proficiency for the education of new public health nurses and for managing the performance of current public health practitioners [3]. All SCPHNs are educated to the new NMC [3] standards and locally programmes in practice and in universities are offering public health education and training, which are developing skills and knowledge in practitioners.

The UK Public Health Skills and Career Framework is a tool developed by the Public Health Resource Unit for describing the skills and knowledge needed across all levels of the public health workforce. It was developed to aid collaboration and coherence across the diverse public health workforce, in order to maximise its collective contribution and underpin the influence of public health in the UK. Wright et al. are reviewing the usefulness of the tool for facilitating a shared approach to strengthening public health competence within and across countries.

Societal trends and the predicted needs of the health care system encourage a focus on community collaboration in an effort to improve the health of communities [50]. Fisher Robertson [50] asserts one of the most sophisticated skills required by health care providers is population health management, which McAlearney (cited in Ref. [50, p. 495]) purports 'involves the use of population-focussed health promotion and disease prevention interventions . . . designed to improve a community's . . . health status in cost effective ways'. It is also argued that a theoretical restructuring of health provision to encapsulate the environment and provide extensive interdisciplinary models of delivery is required [56] along with skills in leadership, responsibility and power being given to front-line practitioners and a financial framework conducive to public health interventions [65].

Ethics of public health

The above dialogue has made the presumption that the state has a responsibility towards reducing ill health and inequalities; reducing the causes of ill health; protecting and promoting the health of children and vulnerable people; helping people avoid unhealthy behaviours and ensuring healthy choices are the easiest choices. However, within these challenges it is also important that public health programmes should:

- Not attempt to coerce adults to lead healthy lives. Yet this is difficult in the working environment where in some workplaces health surveillance is statutory in order to comply with the 1974 Health and Safety at Work Act [67]
- Minimise using any measure without consultation
- Minimise intrusion on personal lifestyle choices

Sir Muir Gray, the chief knowledge officer of the NHS, argues that 'In the 21st century, knowledge is the key element to improving health. In the same way that people need clean, clear water, they have a right to clean, clear knowledge'. At a presentation at the CPHVA conference in 2007 [68], he suggested there are varying issues in the provision of health care in the UK:

- Poor quality of health care
- Waste
- Unknowing variations in policy and practice
- Poor patient experience
- Overenthusiastic adoption of interventions of low value
- Failure to get new evidence into practice
- Failure to manage uncertainty

Surely then the aim of public health nursing practice is to help to overcome these challenges with effective collaboration, planning and engagement with the client groups they serve.

Summary

The NMC standards [3] and the cited literature suggest that SCPHNs require the theoretical skills and practical knowledge to work in community partnerships and interdisciplinary teams; to facilitate change; conduct population and community health needs assessments; develop and improve health promotion and disease prevention programmes; and advocate politically to help communities fulfil their health potential. Despite the barriers and challenges discussed, there are many examples of excellent work and innovation and creativity within public health nursing. However, sustainability of these innovative practices is a concern. Attention to addressing some of the above solutions offered could ensure that innovative work that is based on a preventative and social model of health would be sustainable in the future and achieve a reduction in health inequalities and an improvement in public health and well-being. Questions that remain open to debate and discussion are whether it is actually necessary to have a public health nursing qualification in order to practice effectively as a public health nurse? For OHN and some SN working outside of the NHS, employers may not be that interested in having a public health nurse as long as it is a nurse who can deliver the services they require. However, this can lead to reactive health care provision rather than true proactive health promotion. Truly proactive health promotion can address problems before they occur and working upstream, preventing people jumping into troubled waters, is for many the best place for nurses to be.

References

1 Haycock-Stuart EA. Public health nursing: issues for practice, research and policy. *Community Practitioner* 2004; **77**: 9.

2 Royal College of Nursing. *Defining Nursing.* London: Royal College of Nursing, 2003.

3 Nursing and Midwifery Council. *Standards of Proficiency for Specialist Community Public Health Nurses.* London: Nursing and Midwifery Council, 2004.

4 Turton P. Public health: the professional response. In: Costello J, Haggart M, eds. *Public Health and Society.* Hampshire: Palgrave Macmillan, 2003, pp. 151-69.

5 Butt Y. Accessed June 2006 on www.publichealth.com.

6 Department of Health. *Essence of Care for Health Promotion.* London: HMSO, The Stationery Office, 2006.

7 Elliott L, Crombie IK, Irvine L, Cantrell J, Taylor J. The effectiveness of public health nursing: the problems and solutions in carrying out a review of systematic reviews. *Journal of Advanced Nursing* 2004; **45**(2): 117-25.

8 Coverdale GE, Taylor DP, Elliott R. *Specialist Community Public Health Nursing Degree Course Handbook.* Leeds: Leeds Metropolitan University, 2004.

9 World Health Organization. *Health Promotion Glossary.* Geneva: World Health Organization, 1998.

10 Department of Health. *Making a Difference: A Consultation Paper.* London: HMSO, The Stationery Office, 1998.

11 Department of Health. *Saving Lives - Our Healthier Nation.* London: The Stationery Office, 1999.

12 Department of Health. *Making a Difference: Strengthening the Nursing, Midwifery and Health Visiting Contributions to Health and Healthcare.* London: HMSO, The Stationery Office, 1999.

13 Department of Health. *The NHS Plan - A Plan for Investment, a Plan for Reform.* London: HMSO, The Stationery Office, 2000.

14 Department of Health. *Liberating the Talents: How PCT's and Nurses Can Deliver the NHS Plan.* London: HMSO, The Stationery Office, 2002.

15 Community Practitioners and Health Visitor's Association and Department of Health. *Liberating the Public Health Talents of Community Practitioners and Health Visitors.* London: HMSO, The Stationery Office, 2003.

16 Department of Health. *Choosing Health - Making Healthier Choices Easier.* London: HMSO, The Stationery Office, 2004.

17 Department of Health. *The Chief Nursing Officer's Review of the Nursing, Midwifery and Health Visiting Contribution to Vulnerable Children and Young People.* London: Department of Health, 2004.

18 Department of Health. *Our Health, Our Care, Our Say.* London: HMSO, The Stationery Office, 2006.

19 Department of Health. *School Nurse Practice Development Resource Pack*, Rev. edn. London: HMSO, The Stationery Office, 2006.

20 World Health Organization. *Ottowa Charter for Health Promotion.* First International Conference in Health Promotion, Ottowa. Copenhagen: World Health Organization, 1986.

21 Danielson E, Krogerus-Therman I, Siverston B, Sourtzi P. Nursing and public health in Europe – a new continuous education programme. *International Nursing Review* 2005; **52**: 32-8.

22 Richman J. Holding public health up for inspection. In: Costello J, Haggart M, eds. *Public Health and Society.* Hampshire: Palgrave Macmillan, 2003, pp. 3-21.

23 Scriven A, Orme J. eds. *Health Promotion: Professional Perspectives*, 2nd edn. Hampshire: Palgrave Macmillan, 2001.

24 Coverdale GE, Lancaster K. HNA: the theory practice gap recedes. *Journal of Community Nursing* 2006; **20**(8): 10-16.

25 Hooper J, Longworth P. *Health Needs Assessment in Primary Health Care Workbook*, Version 2. London: Health Development Agency, 1998.

26 National Institute for Clinical Excellence. *Health Needs Assessment – A Practical Guide* (available at www.nice.org.uk). London: Health Development Agency, 2005.

27 Baggott R. *Public Health: Policy and Politics.* London: Routledge, 2000.

28 Kawachi I. Cities that make you sick. In: *UKPHA Conference*, March 2007, Edinburgh, 2007.

29 Nursing and Midwifery Council. *The Nursing and Midwifery Order 2001* (SI 2002/253) (available at www.hmso.gov.uk). Norwich: The Stationery Office, 2001.

30 Nursing and Midwifery Council. *The Code: Standards of Conduct, Performance and Ethics for Nurses and Midwives.* London: Nursing and Midwifery Council, 2008.

31 United Kingdom Central Council. *Standards for Specialist Education and Practice.* London: HMSO, 2001.

32 Council for the Education and Training of Health Visitors (CETHV). *An Investigation into the Principles of Health Visiting.* London: CETHV, 1977.

33 Sir William Beveridge. *Social Insurance and Allied Services Report.* London: HMSO, 1942.

34 Acheson D. *Independent Inquiry into Inequalities in Health.* Accessed November 2003 on http://www.official-documents.co.uk/document/dh/ih/ih.htm; 1998.

35 Wainwright P, Thomas J, Jones M. Health promotion and the role of the school nurse: a systematic review. *Journal of Advanced Nursing* 2000; **32**(5): 1083-91.

36 Madge H, Franklin A. *Change, Challenge and School Nursing.* London: CPHVA, 2003.

37 Lightfoot J, Bines W. Working to keep school children healthy: the complementary roles of school staff and school nurses. *Journal of Public Health Medicine* 2000; **22**(1): 74-80.

38 Tones K, Green J. *Health Promotion: Planning and Strategies.* London: Sage, 2004.

39 Buchanan DR. A new ethic for health promotion: reflections on a philosophy of health education for the 21st century. *Health Education and Behaviour* 2006; **33**(3): 290-304.

40 Laverack G. *Public Health: Power, Empowerment and Professional Practice.* Hampshire: Palgrave Macmillan, 2005.

41 Farmer R, Miller D. *Lecture Notes on Epidemiology and Public Health Medicine*, 3rd edn, Oxford: Blackwell Scientific Publications, 1991.

42 Beaglehole R, Bonita R. Challenges for public health in the global context – prevention and surveillance. *Scandinavian Journal of Public Health* 2001; **29**: 81–3.

43 Bonita R, Beaglehole R, Tord Kjellström. *Basic Epidemiology*. Geneva: World Health Organization, 2006.

44 Williams RR, Hopkins PN, Stephenson S, Wu L, Hunt SC. Primordial prevention of cardiovascular disease through applied genetics. *Preventive Medicine* 1999; **29**(6, Pt 2): S41–9.

45 Department of Children, Schools and Families. *Establishing a Food Partnership*. Accessed on http://www.teachernet.gov.uk/doc/5562/EstablishingFoodPartnership.pdf; 2003.

46 Department of Health. *Report of the Chief Medical Officer's Project to Strengthen the Public Health Function*. London: HMSO, 2001.

47 Elliston K, Wilkinson J. Supporting public health practitioners. *Primary Health Care* 2006; **16**(6): 18–20.

48 Cross S, Block D, LaVohn J, Reckinger D, Olson Keller L, Strohschein S et al. Development of the public health nursing competency instrument. *Public Health Nursing* 2006; **23**(2): 108–14.

49 Coverdale GE. *Public Health Nurses – Fit for Practice*? Research Dissertation, University of Leeds. Pending publication, 2007.

50 Fisher Robertson J. Does advanced community/public health nursing practice have a future? *Public Health Nursing* 2004; **21**(5): 495–500.

51 Croghan E, Johnson C, Aveyard P. School nurses: policies, working practices, roles and value perceptions. *Nursing and Health Care Management and Policy* 2004; **47**(4): 377–85.

52 Grumbach K, Miller J, Mertz E, Finnochio L. How much public health in public health nursing practice? *Public Health Nursing* 2004; **21**(3): 266–76.

53 Yamashita M, Miyaji F, Akimoto R. The public health nursing role in rural Japan. *Public Health Nursing* 2005; **22**(2): 156–65.

54 Plews C, Billingham K, Rowe A. Public health nursing: barriers and opportunities. *Health and Social Care in the Community* 2000; **8**(2): 138–46.

55 McMurray R, Cheater F. Vision, permission and action: a bottom up perspective on the management of public health nursing. *Journal of Nursing Management* 2004; **12**: 43–50.

56 Uosukainen L. Promotion of the good life by public health nurses. *Public Health Nursing* 2001; **18**(6): 375–84.

57 Keleher H. Repeating history? Public and community health nursing in Australia. *Nursing Enquiry* 2000; **7**(4): 258–65.

58 Department of Health and Social Security. *Inequalities in Health: Report of a Research Working Group Chaired by Sir Douglas Black*. London: Department of Health and Social Security, 1980.

59 Acheson D. *Committee of Enquiry into the Future Development of the Public Health Function*. London: HMSO, 1988.

60 Department of Health. *Facing the Future: A Review of the Role of Health Visitor's*. Accessed on www.dh.gov.uk/cno. London: Department of Health, 2007.

61 Dame Carol Black. *Working for a Healthier Tomorrow. A Review of the Health of Britain's Working Age Population*. London: HMSO, The Stationery Office, 2008.

62 Department of Health and Department for Education and Skills. *Looking for a School Nurse*? London: HMSO, The Stationery Office, 2006.

63 Department of Health. *The Tackling Health Inequalities: 2007 Status Report on the Programme for Action.* London: HMSO, 2007.

64 DeBell D, Tomkins AS. *Discovering the Future of School Nursing. The Evidence Base.* London: Amicus, CPHVA, 2006.

65 Baggott R. From sickness to health? Public health in England. *Public Money and Management* 2005; **25**(4): 229-36.

66 Wright J, Rao M, Walker K. The UK public health skills and career framework - could it help to make public health the business of every workforce? *Public Health* 2008; **122**: 541-4.

67 Health and Safety Executive. Health and Safety at Work etc. Act 1974. Accessed 18 August 2008 on http://www.hse.gov.uk/legislation/hswa.pdf; 1974.

68 Sir Muir Gray. CPHVA Conference, Torquay, 2007.

Chapter 3

Theoretical Perspectives of Health Visiting

Faith Muir and Paul Reynolds

Learning objectives

After reading this chapter you will be able to:

- Appreciate the role of the health visitor and identify how practice has evolved
- Understand how the principles of health visiting underpin specialist community public health practice (health visiting)
- Explore health interpretation and need in relation to health inequalities and sustainable health
- Understand the value of health promotion and the health visitor's pivotal role within the community

Introduction

The practice of health visiting is an intimate endeavour requiring insight far in excess of traditional nursing practice; health visitors are privileged, they observe family transition, tradition and change. Effective practice involves public health enablement and collaborative undertakings. Working with and within the community allows health visitors to consolidate their practice and in doing so blend new and existing knowledge, to form the foundations of practical experience. Health visiting is exciting, vibrant, emotional and challenging; moreover, this vibrancy is the dominion of specialist community public health nursing which is the cornerstone of health visiting practice.

Historical perspective

From a historical perspective, health visiting has developed from a personal service into a public health service which incorporates elements of the original role and is reflective of practice today [1, 2].

Manchester and Salford Sanitary Association was founded to contract maternal ignorance and increasing infant mortality in 1862, whereby, Manchester and Salford Ladies Health Society appointed the first health visitor. These women were ideally placed to help and enable women improve their health and well-being, increase their understanding of the importance of childcare in the hope that infant mortality would be reduced significantly [3]. They would visit the poor in their own homes and promote health and hygiene; moreover, this approach provided a unique service that focused on wellness rather than sickness. It is clear that health visitor's main function was dominated by the social events of the industrial revolution. They were first coined as 'sanitary missionaries', ladies who interacted with the public in improving public health education supported by local government at a time when infant mortality was rising, and public health had become increasingly poor as communicable diseases were on the increase. The Public Health Act of 1848 showed interest not only in the nation's health but introduced a means by which this could be addressed. It was clear at this time that health was moving into a new era in relation to health care in this country. Indeed, it was administered with the sole aim of reducing infant mortality but also intended to reform the existing fragmented services [4]. It is clear from the early literature that public health and well-being was at the fore regarding this pioneering venture [5], and eventually the Health Visitors Association was formed in 1896; furthermore, health visiting remains true to its ideology regarding social and public health endeavours. At this time, those appointed as health visitors came from a variety of backgrounds including doctors, nurses and graduates [6]. Historically, prevention and health education proved to be the main focus of public health practice at this time and this was embraced by the newly appointed health visitors. Clearly, it was believed that there was a direct correlation between infant mortality and social conditions, limited education, malnutrition and poverty; in addition, improved health care was dependent upon a collaborative approach including a general awareness raising, an ability to control and treat infection and improve social conditions. The idea of improved family welfare was central to this provision of care [7].

Sanitary women: the way ahead

'Sanitary women' proved beneficial and it was soon realised that the role had great possibility. Nevertheless, it was not until the turn of the century that the potential of health visiting was realised and London was the first borough to formalise a training programme for health visitors' 'sanitary ladies' allowing them to educate families in their own home and in 1914 health visiting was formally recognised. Furthermore, following an Act of Parliament in 1918, the Maternity and Child Welfare Act gave local authorities the power to address welfare work. This resulted in significantly reduced parameters of care and education as health visitors now focused on child health as opposed to family welfare; nevertheless, work undertaken by health visitors across the country proved variable based on local need [8].

The National Health Service (1948): health visiting practice re-considered

The inception of the National Health Service (NHS) in 1948 signified change and the potential of health visiting was re-visited whereby, prevention and family health exploring the social implications of family welfare were reinstated [9]. Progress and development in the field of health visiting moved forward and in 1956 the Jameson Report [10], an enquiry into health visiting practice examined both nursing and health visiting perspectives. The report recommended the setting up of integrated nurse education courses which included both basic nursing and health visiting. The value government placed on health visiting marked a change in direction; moreover, it highlighted current need within society, therefore, a less restrictive practice was favoured which required health visiting practice to be more family centred. Jameson in 1956 described health visiting practice at this time as a means to procure both social and educational support for families in the community.

Health visiting practice arrives, the defining moment

This report [10] was pivotal and as a consequence, the Council for the Training of Health Visitors (CTHVs) was set up which later became the Council for the Education and Training of Health Visitors (CETHVs). The CETHV published a seminal document which defined health visiting training and education [11]; moreover, this document provided the framework for successive re-examinations and remains stoic in its resolve to underpin health visiting [12, 13]. More recently, however, Cowley and Frost [14] have updated the 1992 principles of health visiting [15] to reflect a more contemporary approach to health visitor's public health practice in the twenty-first century.

Health visiting appraisal and organisational change

Health visiting has constantly re-examined and re-evaluated practice and is not without its critics, furthermore, despite criticisms has maintained focus and forbearing [16]. It has been argued that Jameson in 1956 did health visiting a disservice by confusing the role of the social worker and health visitor, suggesting that in an attempt to legitimise the profession the association with nursing was in hindsight a retrograde step [9]. Nonetheless, a state-registered qualification was required as a pre-requisite for health visitor training and in 1962 the CTHV led the way in health visitor education and in subsequent years set new standards of entry establishing courses in higher educational institutes, acknowledging practitioners in their own right [4]. In 1983, the CETHV ceased and its duties were embraced by the United Kingdom Central Council for Nursing, Midwifery and Health Visiting (UKCC) and the four National Boards (England, Northern Ireland, Scotland and Wales) [17-19]. In 1992, the boards were disbanded and restructured [20], whereupon, health visitor training or specialist community health care nursing often referred to as specialist practitioner qualification, became an integral component of the post-registration nursing framework [21]. In addition, the final role of the UKCC was to commission a detailed analysis to establish requirements for pre-registration health visitor education and training. Once completed, this analysis was presented to and accepted by the UKCC (final meeting) in 2002, whereupon, implementation was agreed at the inaugural meeting of the Nursing and Midwifery Council (NMC) in 2002 [14].

Internalising and re-affirming practice is quite a radical perspective; and despite changes, health visiting has always focused upon need and a reduction in health inequality and inequity [22]. What is clear is that this journey does not diminish health visiting practice but strengthens it, and serves to show how integral health visiting practice is to family and community public health [23]; furthermore, health visitors can reach the privileged and the needy within society. This philosophy is engrained into public health practice, which guides and informs current thinking and underpins health visiting practice potential [24], and identifies health visitors as specialist community public health practitioners.

Health visiting in context: the current debate

Health visiting practice is controversial, dynamic and integral to public health; nevertheless, the role has been the cause of much debate resulting in recent reviews [25, 26]. The antecedent to these was the publication of a document re-affirming health visiting practice principles [14] which set the scene for a much improved service in the twenty-first century. However, parallels can be drawn from earlier literature revealing that health visiting practice has continually had to demonstrate its value and worth; here, Twinn [16] engaged the profession in a judicious debate responding to Goodwin [27] who suggested health visiting practice had become methodical and prescriptive. Arguably, any process that questions professional practice is contentious [28] and this provides a timely reminder that the dilemma experienced by the health visiting profession today is contiguous and needs to be addressed.

Health visitor's public health role: a concept of practice

Public health is by its very nature capricious and health visitors have responded accordingly and in spite of known fragilities with regard to role clarity. In response, health visitors have acquired the skill and knowledge which has led to academic, educational and professional fulfilment. Health visitors in the twenty-first century need to continue and consolidate this learning of worth to secure and produce 'situation knowledge', undertake practice evaluation, engage in research and publish the findings. This educational progression is both valued and recognised and will provide structure to support practice development; moreover, it will improve role transparency and engender a personal and professional satisfaction. It could be argued that health visitors could become a passive observant of their own demise if this interaction does not occur; such is the enormity of the health visiting contribution to public health in the twenty-first century [14]. Responsible health visiting requires po-litically astute health visitors who can actively respond to public health needs; engage in health visiting/health visitor development, and embrace collabo-rative public health endeavours to secure health improvements and address health inequalities [14, 29]. In addition, role continuance requires active and proactive and political health visitors who regard research and education as pivotal to health visiting success to secure their future development in the public health arena.

Furthermore, health visiting is an investment in the future; it is sustainable, responsive and significantly contributes to society's health and well-being by working with and within communities [30]. This is health visitor's strength, the ability to identify and respond to the needs, demands and challenges of the community and to stimulate and create new directions in practice [14].

New directions: a focus for research

Health visitors are a valuable commodity and proponents of health visiting practice recognise their value within public health and health promotion [25]. As discussed previously, health visitors have the capacity to ameliorate the known causes of conflict, clarify their role and reduce the likelihood of pro-fessional ambivalence towards them [31]. Health visitors have the capability to realise support through practice endeavours and research into practice. Reciprocity and trust from allied professionals is fundamental if effective health visiting practice is to be realised. Also, health visitors have to recog-nise disparity within their own profession if collaborative relationships are to improve; moreover, increasing competency, proficiency and skill will facilitate this change and reduce role confusion.

Cowley and Frost [14] define health visiting in terms of activities which are proactive to address need that is both recognised and unrecognised. Similarly, Twinn [16] suggested that health visiting was identified specifically through domains such as individual, environmental, psychological and emancipatory; clearly, this quorate approach reinforces and underpins the principles estab-lished in 1977 [11], re-defined by Twinn and Cowley [15] and invigorated by Cowley and Frost [14]. This grounded approach to health visiting remains apposite and vital. The principles remain vibrant, and distinguished, placing health visiting in a pivotal position at the centre of public life, focusing on com-munity, charged with the responsibility to ensure the public's health potential is realised and sustained.

Extending the boundaries

The principles of health visiting: the mantra of health visiting practice

- The search for health needs
- The stimulation of an awareness of health needs
- The influence on policies affecting health
- The facilitation of an awareness of health needs

> ### Activity 3.1
>
> Take time to read and consider the principles in their entirety. This philosophy embraced by health visitors is fundamental to all their public health practice. A broader and more enduring understanding will enable you to challenge and consider the importance of policy, practice and research.

Health visiting review

A review of the role of health visitors [25] placed the principles at the fore once again and set out clearly defined structures to further frame and consolidate health visiting practice in the twenty-first century. This document defined the perpetual change within society and provided a health visiting response to parallel these needs evidenced within society reflecting the valuable contribution health visitors can make to improve the public's health. The parameters and scope of practice are specific and public health improvement remains pivotal in all work undertaken by health visitors. Clearly, this aspect of a health visitor's role is unique and sets it apart from any other professional group working in the community and this has been further underpinned in this document. There remains an even greater emphasis upon research, publishing and evidence-based practice to inform best practice, policies to strengthen future practice and emphasis on a universal service set within a targeted service framework. This document acknowledges the changes within society, such as family structure, increasing diversity, excluded families and children, a greater emphasis is placed upon vulnerability, minorities within minorities, changing environments and public expectation. In addition, the document acknowledges this diversity and emphasises that the health visiting service will contribute significantly and endeavour to meet those needs both professionally and collaboratively. The integrity of the profession has been realised and the potential acknowledged; moreover, the government's response [26] suggests that health visiting will play a vital role in shaping the public's health and play a key role in tackling the social determinants of health and improve health and well-being.

Improved public health, health education and health promotion is the essence of health visiting practice [14]. The Darzi Report [30] further consolidates the role of community practitioners and recognises the need for improved care and quality within the NHS; furthermore, the report highlighted a collaborative approach to public health improvements and development, suggesting that an empowered workforce can deliver and sustain the most important elements of public health practice relying on nurses, midwives and health visitors to deliver that care and improve well-being. Inequalities in health care remain the focus for all primary and community health care practitioners; furthermore [24], if inequalities are to be addressed then it is vital that health visitors re-establish their priorities and consolidate practice of work to ensure the principles are adhered to and underpin all future work. Highlighting need and unmet need remains an essential attribute of public health practice and is engrained within the health visiting role. Health visitors working with and within the community ensure that the wider determinants that affect health, inequity and inequality are addressed.

The correlation between the rhetoric and practice of health visiting

The health needs agenda is and remains the focus of public health practice [32]. Health visitors are required to embrace this philosophy and apply the rhetoric from a community perspective. This emphasis on a traditional approach to health visiting (universal service) in the formative years enables health visitors to prioritise their work and manage their workload. Ostensibly, health visitors have profiled their areas in an attempt to clarify their work but also to highlight need and unmet need within an area. Getting to know your patch is certainly one of the most fundamental components of a health visitor's role; without an accurate picture of the community setting or geographical area, the needs of the community cannot be fully realised or assessed [33]. Public health measures including mortality and morbidity figures and the demographics are an essential part of practice; however, these may only reflect key areas of need and may not truly represent the community as a whole [34]. This is not to say that the information is not accurate; nonetheless, they may only serve to show determinants that have targeted and quality of life issues may go unchecked. This unmet need from a population perspective is a key area of public health practice and requires a collaborative approach if society's health is to be improved and sustained [35].

Community health visiting

The principles of health visiting provide a framework and underpin all work undertaken in the community and are comparable to the public health agenda [14]; moreover, it is becoming increasingly important to recognise that no one professional group can tackle the ills of society, and health visitors must engage and seek out others in the community to further and sustain community working to improve outcomes that are measurable and evaluative [36].

Public health is central to health visiting practice; therefore, it is important to consider how health is experienced and expressed in order to understand what influences choice and how best to facilitate and enable families and communities to engage with their health. Part of this process is being aware of what inhibits change and limits choices [24]. The wider social determinants of health contribute to health choices and this knowledge provides health visitors with a much broader capacity to engage with families and communities and to understand how change can be achieved.

Clearly, it is important that health visitors and health visiting practice reflect the diversity of the population it serves by providing dynamic and proactive health initiatives to engage with an ever-increasing public expectation. Integral to this is providing new and innovative ways of addressing need which can be far reaching and complex [37]. Health visitors need to clearly understand their role and how the principles frame practice, justify and defend the health requirements of their community and contribute to the wider social and political determinants that pervade public life [38].

Health visitors are ideally placed to ensure that all children and families receive optimum health promotion and guidance at specific times, for example, throughout a child's formative years and when dealing with vulnerable groups within society. Child development potential needs to be seen from a broader perspective in terms of sustainability; furthermore, surveillance has been replaced by the child health promotion programme [39, 40] which facilitates a broader capacity to engage in child health education [41]. Health visiting has the capability to tackle the problems faced by society today if the principles of health visiting [14] can be facilitated and coordinated across a broader spectrum exploring intersectoral, collaborative, partnership working. Furthermore, health visitors have the skill and knowledge to engage and deliver improved care once need has been identified.

Defining community

In order to apply the principles in practice [14] the health visitor must identify what community means to them.

Activity 3.2

What does community mean to you? Consider this statement and take time to reflect upon your response before continuing.

Community is a place that is identifiable and familiar, a place where we belong but equally it may be somewhere we dislike and wish to move away from. Skidmore [42] suggested that community could be deemed a myth, whereby society had been conditioned to think there is a shared identity and purpose. Arguably, the notion of community suggests coherence and collaboration but these are just words to identify a location, one that could be fragmented and disagreeable. Putnam [43] explores in depth the notion of a shared identity, communities and discusses commonalities of reciprocity and identifiable collegiate goals as a means to improve health and well-being. Community is by its very nature diverse, evolving, and as such the known dynamics can change and the landscape alter, but what is important to realise is that the community is made up of people, individuals, families, groups and organisations; collectively, they are termed 'community'. In theory, communities include everyone, infants, young people, those in midlife, the old and vulnerable within society; however, communities include the socially excluded and mentally ill and the disadvantaged which is a far more realistic representation of a community [44]. In addition, community is a geographical area, a shared environment or region; however, community may only reflect a similarity of space.

Forging links with the community is an integral part of health visiting practice, and in an attempt to promote and engage with the health and health needs of this diverse population group the complexities of 'community' must be understood.

How does community equate to health visiting practice?

Health visitors work in a variety of areas (settings).
These could include:

- Geographical
- General practitioner (GP) attached
- Corporate
- Urban area
- Rural area
- Hospital based
(other areas include prisons, mother and baby units, refuges, hostels and homeless shelters).

Health visitors work with and allied to other professional groups in and within the community. If we look at the GP-attached health visitor in a rural setting you are more likely to work closely with the practice nurse, school nurse, social worker, community psychiatric nurse, midwife, GP, practice manager, community paediatrician, speech and language therapist and learning disability nurse (this list is not exhaustive).

You may have responsibility towards the under five/four population and their families, antenatal commitment, mother and baby clinic, rural outreach clinics, postnatal support groups, child health promotion, health promotion sessions for families and elderly groups (to name a few). As a health visitor, you may have a specialist interest in child protection (in addition to your normal caseload), you may be involved in a domestic abuse forum (or a refuge if one is in your area), you may be on the local council medical committee, meet regularly with social services and be involved in other collaborative endeavours to promote health and well-being in your community and/or new initiatives in your area to address health inequalities, need and perception of need. Some examples could include (a safe play area, teenage mothers or parenting support, improved housing or access to counsellors; similarly, you may want to improve existing services). In order to understand need consideration must be given to the lay perspective of health.

The lay perspective of health: a health visiting view

Health interpretation is variable as it means different things to different people. Firstly, it is worthwhile considering what health means to you.

> ### Activity 3.3
>
> How would you define health? Consider this from a personal and professional perspective. Take time to reflect upon this.

Most of us would concede that being healthy refers to the fact that we are 'fit and well' and have no medically defined illness. Arguably, the term 'health' could be considered as abstract, and is a concept that requires further scrutiny. Blaxter [45] suggests that the way in which we experience the world reflects our interpretation of it; moreover, reflecting on work undertaken by Foucault, she argues that perception is a systematic social discourse which is by definition subjective. In addition, she cites studies which infer that health interpretation is based on gender, age and social class. Laverack [46] supports this claim suggesting that multiple interpretations are reflective of both personal and cultural experience. In addition, he goes on to cite work by Labonte [47] reinforcing the complexities of interpretation stating that self-esteem impacts on definition; moreover, health can also be viewed as functional, in so much as persons may have a disease (diabetes mellitus), for example, yet regard themselves as fit and able. What is clear is that health is experienced in differing ways and interpretation is representative of 'real life experiences' irrespective of culture, ethnicity, gender or race [36]. Furthermore, it is important to realise that health interpretation reflects a far more diverse, complex and enduring problem which needs to be carefully appraised. In addition, health interpretation can be viewed as relative and absolute [48], reinforcing cultural belief and experience. In conclusion, health is personal and cannot be separated from the experience.

> ### Activity 3.4
>
> What can influence health interpretation? Consider this sentence and write down what you consider is important and provide a rationale.

The important thing to remember is that despite all the rhetoric that surrounds health interpretation, health is a political issue because of the health divide, inequality and inequity [24]. Health is a resource and has a cost and therefore, good health is dependent upon political will and determination; moreover, political intervention can in part remedy the inequalities that exist by targeting the social determinants of health which requires political action [49]. As cited earlier, improved access to services, improved housing, safe play and activities for children and adolescents, health is not just about improving screening uptakes and providing immunisations; it is about quality of life and improving lifestyles which impacts on health outcomes [50]. Stress and the predisposition to mental health, employment opportunity, improved nutrition in early life, work-life balance, transport and road safety; all of these are politically driven and can significantly contribute to the entitlement of good health prospects [51].

Meeting unmet need and what this actually means: a health visiting perspective

Activity 3.5

How would you best describe need? What characteristics do you think are integral to need and how can these be justified from a health visiting perspective?

Need is an ambiguous word and it is not unlike health in its interpretation [33]. Need conjures up all kinds of thoughts to suggest we understand the concept. We may think of need in terms of material objects; however, this could be deemed as a requirement and not necessarily reflect need. We all need food and water, the basics to sustain life, and material possessions may be considered desirable but not necessary or needed to survive. Need is therefore a relative concept requiring a more in-depth appraisal to underpin and direct health visiting practice and effectively tackle disparities in health [52].

As discussed earlier, need has been described as a necessity without which human life could not be sustained [44]; therefore, consideration must be given to basic needs and how to differentiate between essential and social needs. Maslow [53] (see Box 3.1) attempted to distinguish need in terms of essential elements and likened need to a hierarchal system, starting with physiological needs being addressed first which would enable the individual to progress; moreover, each individual need would have to be satisfied in order to progress to the next stage and so on (to achieve self-actualisation).

Box 3.1   Maslow hierarchy of need

(5) Self-actualisation
(4) Esteem needs ↑
(3) Belongingness and love needs ↑
(2) Safety needs ↑
(1) Physiological (essential needs, i.e. shelter, water and food)

Adapted from Maslow [53].

The complexity of need is explored here in more detail by Bradshaw [54]. This taxonomy of need is divided into four (**normative, felt, expressed** and **comparative**), reflecting both the individual and population expectation of health and the capacity to change. *Examples cited reflect health visiting practice*:

Normative need: It is generally agreed that normative need is categorised by a professional, for example there may be some safety issues in a home which the professional feels requires attention. A good example of this would be the absence of a fireguard and the associated risk. The procurement of a fireguard is a desired outcome (a need) to prevent accidental injury. You could argue that it is a valued judgement on behalf of the professional involved; however, child safety is paramount and the family may not have the necessary funds. Clearly, this area of practice is fraught with difficulty; yet, the professional in their opinion feels a guard is needed.

Felt need: Felt need differs from normative need as it is instigated by an individual, family or group and not a professional and can be equated with want. Felt need and expectation are inextricably linked and often perceived as need. An example of this could be when a parent's perception of care differs with that of the professional; they may feel they need more help. Here an expectation or a want is confused with a need. This felt need can be at a variance with what is actually available and this can cause problems for the professional; furthermore, this type of need is relative.

Expressed need: This is when a felt need becomes a demand. An example could be a request for a housing letter as a family wants a property with more bedrooms and a garden. This expressed need is when a felt need translates into a desire.

Comparative need: This is when individuals, families or groups do not receive the same level of care and they feel there is a disparity. This can sometimes be seen when you compare similar groups in rural and urban areas. The agreed standard falls short and there is a need.

What is evident is 'need' will be interpreted in different ways by professionals, lay people and organisations. Clearly, tensions exist and the definition of need requires a more holistic approach to encapsulate the social, environmental and political determinants of health needs assessment. Part of the health visitor's role is to address need and unmet need in their community but in order to do this, health visitors must be cognisant of health interpretation if identified need is to prove meaningful; obviously, lay perception is key to determining how health and well-being are perceived by the population or community. Public health is central to health visiting practice; therefore, it is important to consider how health is experienced, what influences choice and how best to facilitate and enable families and communities to engage with their health. Part of this process is being aware of what inhibits change and limits choices [55]. The wider social determinants of health contribute to health choices and this knowledge provides health visitors with a much broader capacity to engage with families and communities and to understand how change can be achieved [24]. Clearly, the level of need and unmet need will reflect the diversity of the community and direct practice and this will provide the focus for practice, increase ownership and will enable health visitors to reconnect to the community.

Determinants of health

These are a variety of factors that can inhibit or promote health; they include personal, economic and environmental factors. As stated earlier, factors that influence health and well-being impact significantly on outcomes and can reduce or restrict choice. Dahlgren and Whitehead [56] (Box 3.2) suggested that certain factors exist that are inevitable such as gender and age; however, social, cultural, lifestyle and economic position may be variable but are modifiable. How each of these influences one another has been examined extensively in the literature. However, Davies and Macdowall [48] conclude that each individual determinant is significant and can vary at each stage of all our lives; moreover, interactions between the determinants can impact on health outcomes.

Box 3.2   Determinants

General socioeconomic, cultural and environmental conditions

- Agriculture and food production
- Work environment
- Living and working conditions
- Unemployment
- Water and sanitation
- Health care services
- Housing

Social and community networks
Individual lifestyle factors
Age, sex and hereditary factors

Adapted from Dahlgren and Whitehead [56].

Activity 3.6

Health and childhood nutrition: Make brief notes on why nutrition is important in childhood and how this can impact on health outcomes? Do any other determinants influence choice, and consider what influences our understanding of health. Remember, health, its interpretation and perceptions are personal.

Nutrition can significantly affect health outcomes. Improving infant nutrition is one of the most important determinants of health and development. An inappropriate or inadequate diet in childhood can significantly affect health in later life. Socially disadvantaged families are more likely to feed their children inadequate diets; however, the rise in obesity suggests that prevalence may also be due to environmental and social factors too (see Chapter 1).

Health visiting diaries: what health visitors need to know

Health visitors' public health potential

The concept of public health has been open to scrutiny and interpretation; yet, it is widely accepted that public health refers to a collective collaboration engendered to improve and facilitate the health and well-being of the population. Therefore, public health can be defined as an attempt to improve the functioning and longevity of populations [57]. The Department of Health [50] supports this notion and goes on to suggest that good health and the potential of healthier outcomes are inextricably linked to lifestyle, opportunities for health gain and the way in which people live their lives. Furthermore, health improvement has been linked to many factors such as improved standards of living, better education, enhanced nutrition and housing. This aspect of public health as the primary focus of all intervention parallels the ideology of change that was so vigorously challenged to control and treat infectious diseases, raise educational and economic standards in order to reduce the numbers of premature deaths in the 1860s [58]. Arguably, the nature of the illness may have changed but the primary focus of public health remains the same: to improve and sustain the quality of that life. Nevertheless, the breadth and complexity of public health could be considered a weakness as attempts are made to improve the quality of the population's health by adopting a blame culture inferring that unhealthy activity is avoidable without considering the ramifications of social factors that may inhibit choice or make life more tolerable. Such is the complexity of public health that it is clear, as with health visiting, some groups may consider problems within society in differing ways [59]; therefore, consideration must be given to such opinions and considered accordingly [37].

Health promotion: a health visiting endeavour

Health promotion is seen as the central focus of public health [60, 61] and a means to improve and sustain health. The Ottawa Charter [60] stated that health is a resource for everyday living and the Bangkok Charter [61] reaffirmed this stating that good health is a fundamental right without discrimination. Improving health potential and promoting healthier lifestyles requires political will and innovative health visitors.

Health visiting practice recognises the validity of sustainability, empowerment as cited in the Ottawa Charter and this endeavour is upheld within health visiting philosophy [14]. Moreover, addressing health inequality is the focus of all health visiting practice and social determinants remain the cornerstone of needs assessment in practice [62]. Furthermore, the terms *health promotion* and *health education* have been used synonymously without a clear understanding; therefore, clarity is required [63]. Health education is viewed as the process involved in providing information to facilitate change and by design facilitate improved health. This is usually undertaken on an individual basis requiring partnership and a willingness to engage, an enablement process, but it is also an essential attribute of health promotion. Health promotion, however, explores the concept and risk associated with lifestyles, health behaviour and the broader determinants that impinge on health and health choices such as deprivation, unemployment, poor or inadequate housing, education and diet [48]. In many ways it is not unlike health in its interpretation as is difficult to define. Furthermore, health promotional activity is politically and socially driven; challenging, encompassing public health policy, culture, environmental and social issues in contemporary society [64].

Activity 3.7

Improving the public's health is high on the political agenda. Social, economic and environmental factors can have an enduring effect upon health and deepen health inequalities. Consider current practice and how this is influenced by policy.

Health promotion is by its very nature interwoven and complex; therefore, health promotional activities can be expressed in many ways (a health visiting perspective):

- Individual (mental health and well-being; child health promotion)
- Group (women's health; mental health awareness; teenage mothers; local campaigns to improve awareness of domestic abuse)
- Broader public health campaigns (improving access to services for isolated groups)
- Population health (smoking ban; safer sex; immunisations)

Health promotion in primary care focuses on the social, environmental and economic factors. To summarise, health promotion is a phrase that can be used interchangeably with terms such as health education, health protection, health enhancement and health maintenance [35]. Health promotion is all of these but more specifically it is a means to achieve optimum health.

The challenge of health promotion: health visiting practice

Assessing need in primary care can be challenging. Some of the evidence does not reflect the true nature of incidence as numbers may be too small; similarly, areas have been assessed collectively which is not representative of need and fails to identify pockets of deprivation and/or inequality [35]. Often, figures presented are the ones that are easily identifiable and not necessarily reflective of unmet need. Difficulties arise in measuring the unmeasurable such as continuity and effective communication.

Activity 3.8

Therefore, health visitors must consider: how can you measure effective health promotion in the short term [65]? What mechanisms do you have in place to assess and evaluate practice?

In order to plan and engage in any type of health promotional activity a full assessment of need is required as a pre-requisite to enable services to be targeted appropriately [66], being mindful that the aspiration is good health and the predisposition to poorer health and disease is determined primarily by socioeconomic and environmental influences [24]. Resultant behaviour is often as a consequence of this and determined by the perception of need, health potential and an understanding of enablement, and influential external forces such as the determinants of health. Health promotion is therefore an integral component of public health and improved health gain, one which health visitors need to be mindful of [67]. Clearly, it is important that health visitors and health visiting practice reflect the diversity of the population it serves by providing dynamic and proactive health initiatives to engage with an ever-increasing public expectation. Integral to this is providing new and innovative ways of addressing need which can be far reaching and complex. Health visitors need to clearly understand their role and how the principles frame practice, justify and defend the health requirements of their community and contribute to the wider social and political determinants that pervade public life.

Health visiting in action: the ability to reflect – a mirror for practice

Reflection is an integral part of health visiting practice as it allows practitioners to internalise experiences and explore them in more depth [68]. Reflection also facilitates change and can consolidate practice experience. Furthermore, reflection is an antecedent to improve practice. Reflection is something most people do regularly, it is inevitable and it can have a positive or a negative influence. The ability to internalise and disseminate practice, however, is what sets it apart from other reflective episodes [69]. Reflection is the causal link between theory, practice and growth in a professional field [70]. Health visitors need to be able to critically reflect in order to defend and justify actions, utilising research to underpin practice and sometimes internalise ethical decisions or dilemmas. Specialist practitioners (student health visitors) are required to reflect independently, collectively and openly in order to facilitate change and demonstrate progression and understanding. Reflection can appear superficial, yet it opens up potential and possibility. Reflection is also an enabling process when challenges or limitations in practice require further scrutiny [71]. To summarise, health visitors need to challenge and promote, defend and articulate decisions and substantiate actions regularly; moreover, health visitors are advocates and as such must adhere to the NMC [72] code of professional conduct requiring them to be accountable for practice; therefore, reflection is both challenging and worthwhile.

The concept of empowerment: the *raison d'être* of health promotion

The four principles of health visiting reflect health visiting practice and incorporate the premise of empowerment as a central theme [14]. Working in partnership with and within the community, health visitors enable and empower individuals, communities and groups to engage in their own health [73]. The potential of an empowered community is far reaching and adheres to the assertion laid down in the Ottawa Charter [60] and reaffirmed in the Bangkok Charter [61]. Increasingly, the discussion and research surrounding the notion of empowered individuals and communities suggests that this is more effective if health potential is to be realised [74]. Advocacy and self-empowerment through enablement parallels partnership working and collaborative endeavours; moreover, increasing community knowledge and supporting healthy campaigns underpins the empowerment philosophy enabling the potential of change to be realised [75]. Confidence, knowledge empowerment, partnership and collaborative initiatives are cyclical requiring support and resources to engender improved healthy outcomes [46].

Empowerment is central to health promotion and was defined in the Ottawa Charter [60, p. 1] 'as the process of enabling people to increase control over, and to improve, their health'. Part of this declaration included the idea of 'realising aspirations', 'satisfying needs' and 'health should be seen as a resource for everyday life and not necessarily the object of living.'

Irrespective of health promotional endeavours, the concept of empowerment is difficult to define; moreover, it is often easier to discuss powerlessness than empowerment. Similarly, to empower an individual or group one has to assume there is a desire to be empowered or the capacity to be empowered is present [76]. Self-determination is a key element to empowerment and is fundamental to health promotional policies [77]; moreover, individuals and/or groups will only become empowered if they have the desire to change and it is viewed as a realistic goal. Furthermore, parallels can be drawn from Maslow's [53] hierarchical framework of need when we consider empowerment strategies, antecedents such as desire, capacity and a willingness to change are central to the empowerment process [78]. This ability to change and become empowered may be a gradual process and not necessarily the outcome itself; therefore, in order to achieve the ideal state of empowerment, individuals, groups and communities must be cognisant of the benefits, explore the rationale and engage in the process to actualise health improvement that is sustainable and transparent [46]. In addition, Laverack [46] suggests that practitioners and people must work together if empowerment is to be realised, and suggests that the transformative use of power by practitioners makes the link. Clearly, disparity is inevitable and multifarious; in addition, measuring empowerment is formidable, yet possible; nonetheless, limitations may endure due to culture, race, gender and education (to name a few), but more importantly, health visitors must consider how practice can overcome such challenges or barriers which may inhibit the empowerment potential [79].

An understanding of health promotional models: the application of theory

Health improvement as part of health promotion uses models and approaches to enable and facilitate improved health, moreover, guides the potential development of health promotional activities. These models are based upon a medical approach, behavioural change, social change, empowerment theory and educational improvement [80]. The key principle is the model provides the framework essential to determine behaviour and decision making; therefore, models have evolved from health psychology and the study of human behaviour. Models are a change agent requiring collaboration and partnership if the outcomes are to prove favourable [48]. From a practical point of view these models are inextricably linked, share common features and aspirations; moreover, they are principally determined by their use of language which can be quite confusing [37]. In essence, health visiting has focused upon an applied approach in practice, which reflects the philosophy of health promotion in action. Health promotion explores health potential, embraces the perspective of equity, for that reason, models are a figurative expression or an abstract of change that can address need and direct action to improve health; additionally, a model is a construct to examine and explain outcomes that can be evaluated [36].

Clearly, health promotion encompasses a variety of activities involving individuals, groups, organisations, communities and nations; yet, sometimes confusion remains regarding their application in primary care. Specific models have been used to tackle individual and/or group approaches to behaviour change, an example of their usage is in smoking cessation adapting the stages of change model [81]; however, in order to gain a deeper and more enduring understanding of models health visitors must engage more in their usage. As cited previously, models are not rigid structures, they can and have been adapted in order to best reflect the needs of individual groups, communities etc., what they do provide is a realistic representation of the potential of partnership working required to effectively promote and evaluate health outcomes. In Activity 3.9, there are some examples of models used by health visitors and adapted for health promotional activities.

Activity 3.9

Further reading on models is recommended: Have a look at the following texts in the library or carry out a search on the net: **health belief model** [82]; **stages of change model** [81]; **theory of reasoned action** [83]; **social cognitive theory** [84].

The prospect and scope of health visiting: an assessment of health and inequalities

The assessment of need in a community can be undertaken by all professionals working collaboratively; however, in real terms new or newly appointed health visitors need to be cognisant of the 'population', existing health services, mortality and morbidity data, current infrastructure and resources including all proposed and future health planning (a considerable amount of this information can be accessed from the Annual Report of the Director of Public Health in your area and Primary Care Trusts). In order to truly understand recognised and unrecognised need, health visitors must ensure this process is re-visited (if a profile already exists), or reinstate (if absent). The Annual Report of the Director of Public Health and Census Data will provide insight into current health trends, include success and inequity in your area/region and social configuration; but as cited earlier, this may not reflect the true diversity of your community and practitioners need to be mindful of this [35]. Often, data are limited or difficult to record particularly in rural or hard to reach groups; therefore, what this report will do is provide the primary focus for your initial foray. In some areas the type of information may only reveal what is measurable and may not reflect small pockets of deprivation, inequity or disparity; therefore, it may be difficult to draw any conclusions. This type of practice avoids assumptions and rhetoric, moreover, attempts to improve health for all. Clearly, profiling creates opportunities for further scrutiny. Addressing local health needs (community), by demonstrating an awareness of unrecognised and recognised need is an integral part of health visiting practice and reflects government's policy for improved health opportunities [14]. A community profile will enable you to frame and define your practice area, highlight inequality and help you to construct a community 'picture', which will allow you to start thinking about health visiting practice objectives and more importantly, adheres to the principle of evidence-based practice [85].

Social capital: the myth of a collective and cohesive partnership

Social capital is not a new phenomenon; however, its prominence is now central to public health, health visiting and health policy to ensure the health and well-being of individuals, families, groups and communities are realised and maintained [86]. Social capital is referred to as social interaction, social cohesiveness, connectivity, group membership, including the shared norms of reciprocity and trust, including, formal and informal social networks in and within communities [87]. This current interest has been attributed to the work of Robert Putnam [43] who initially explored the concept of social capital in Italy. Putnam suggested that a society that has no shared identity or common beliefs or goals has limited health potential; therefore, by improving social capital within communities by increasing levels of connectivity using social networks, they were more likely to have improved health gains [88]. This social connectivity significantly affects the health of all members of the community; it is the 'glue' that connects people and communities together, affording protection against the adverse effects of poverty and deprivation. Putnam argued that factors that contributed to poor health gain included communities with little or no social support, fewer social networks, included fragmented and isolated families, increasing social mobility, leaving in its wake isolated groups, with little or no interest in the community and its surrounding areas. In conclusion, such factors contribute to the social decline of a community and this spiralling effect engenders indifference, apathy, negativity and ultimately social exclusion [24].

Putnam [43] has been criticised, suggesting that this utopia of a caring community is unobtainable and fails to consider ethnic and cultural disparity and class differences which can limit the potential for cohesion [89]. Nevertheless, social capital cannot be ignored as a positive health measure in an increasingly isolated society where poverty and deprivation, vulnerability and exclusion, inequality and inequity are prevalent [90]. The potential benefits of collaborative endeavours, participation and social networking in communities can never be underestimated and can have a significant impact on health and well-being [91]; therefore, the concept of social capital and connectivity is certainly a worthy aspiration in community health visiting practice.

Poverty and child health: the myriad of health visiting

Poverty and child health is not far from our conscience on a daily basis and as health visitors we need to explore this concept in more detail in an attempt to understand the ramifications for health visiting practice [92].

Activity 3.10

Do children have choices? Does poverty mean deprived? Think about these questions for a couple of minutes before you continue reading. What do you read in the papers or hear on the news about poverty? Consider your experiences to date.

Poverty is an international problem and needs to be considered in the context of the experience [93, 94]. Poverty is subjective and it is political. Poverty and social deprivation significantly contribute to ill health and a reduction in life expectancy [24]. Poverty is defined as absolute or relative [95]. Absolute poverty is seen as an inability to provide the basics of life, food, clothing, housing and heating; whereas, relative poverty is a perception of inequality based upon society's norms. Living in a deprived area, being unemployed, having poor or inadequate housing, limited education or educational opportunities; disability and the prevalence of mental health all significantly contributes to deprivation and health inequality [90]. Clearly, poverty is a lived experience with no boundaries with any one solution; moreover, the social and economic divide between the rich and poorer members of society are increasing and health inequity between such groups remains. The health of the poorest has improved; however, the health of the more affluent members in society has increased, escalating the health divide still further [96].

Health visitors need to be mindful of the ramifications of deprivation and poverty and its strain on family life [97, 98]. In order to realise their potential, health visitors must concede that despite their best efforts, change takes time and often practice outcomes do not reflect work undertaken and evaluation is not factored into practice [99].

Child health promotion: health visiting opportunities

Child health promotion and child protection is a significant part of health visiting practice and a central component of public health policy and practice. Promoting child health, child mental health [100] and welfare involves government legislation and national policy, as well as health resources at community level [41]. Partnership working is an essential attribute of public health practice and reflects the principles of health visiting. Partnership working involves individuals, families, communities and allied agencies. The Ottawa Charter [60] frames all child health and welfare; furthermore, the National Service Framework for Children, Young People and Maternity Services (Children's NSF) [39, 101] and Every Child Matters (ECM) [102] acknowledge the enduring nature of child and adolescent health and health potential. Essential to health visiting practice is the adherence to the children's NSF [101] and ECM [102]; moreover, contributing to improved child services and care is a pivotal role of practice and this is underpinned by the principles of health visiting practice [14]. Poverty and the risks associated with deprivation provide a platform for health visiting practice, as is an awareness of the social and economic factors that significantly limit and reduce choice; working with families and communities to protect children and increase their health opportunities is integral to the health visiting philosophy.

Activity 3.11

Families that endure poverty and who have limited educational opportunity would benefit from health visitor intervention. Consider this statement and make notes. Reflect on your current experience and practice; consider Dahlgren and Whiteheads framework again [56]. Think about the relationship between poverty and child health. Are families who are disadvantaged limited still further and what can health visitor's do to reduce/limit inequalities and improve child welfare and is this a realistic expectation of practice?

Public health policy: the reality of health visiting practice

Public health policy is designed to improve the public's health and in doing so has focused attention on key aspects of health and health improvement [50]. The government has produced a comprehensive health agenda to reduce health inequalities for the twenty-first century. *Saving Lives: Our Healthier Nation* [103], this provided the foundation for an improved service and better health care. A report commissioned by the government, Wanless [96] reinforced the value of engaging the public in health choices, stating that health care provision would be more cost-effective and success more likely if society were to be more fully engaged; furthermore, he criticised time spent on analysing problems rather than focusing on practical solutions. Choosing health [50] adhered to this participatory theme, acknowledging a need for greater public involvement (engagement) in changing lifestyle. In addition, this paper argued that disadvantaged and marginalised groups within society must be provided with opportunities to make health changes to improve their health, formally acknowledging that inequalities determine health choices, reflecting a far more realistic representation of the realities of life. Choosing health [50] refers to sustainable and cost-effective health care, arguing that existing problems require a fresh approach; furthermore, disparity in health is increasing despite current measures, therefore new and more innovative ways of engaging the public and delivering health care must be considered by health visitors.

Choosing health [50] describes some of the following as 'pointers' for future health care practice:

- A reduction in smoking (biggest preventable cause of ill health)
- Improved sexual health awareness and a reduction in sexually transmitted diseases (Chlamydia, which can cause infertility)
- Improvements in mental health problems, focusing on young people
- A reduction in the number of suicides, the commonest cause of death in males under 35 years of age
- Improving nutrition and a reduction in obesity

The White Paper, 'Our health, our care, our say' [51] recommends collaborative endeavours to improve health, proposing health and social care initiatives, improved educational opportunities and improved services to poorer areas to close the health divide. Meeting the needs of the local community (in local settings) is the main focus of this paper, overseen by Directors of Public Health. This paper embraces the ideology of Our Healthier Nation [103], Wanless [96] and Choosing Health [50], building on current services and promoting health and well-being locally, suggesting health promotion should be integrated and responsive in nature and certainly an integral part of health visiting practice.

'Our health, our care, our say' [51] explores the potential of:

- Health promotion and education (prevention)
- Improved access to health and social care
- Increased community services
- Needs-based care
- Increased parity of services

Clearly, the role of government is to improve access to services and the quality of that care, furthermore, create opportunities through collaborative endeavours and partnership working. To affect change, health visitors have a vital role to play, none more so than working with communities to facilitate improved health opportunities and actively seek out unrecognised need in their area [14]. Facilitating the potential for change in individuals, groups and communities enables and creates opportunity for health gain and reflects the philosophy of health visiting.

Activity 3.12

Think about current policy. Health visitors need to consider what changes need to be made and how change could be achieved. Get involved in local organisations, and community groups. If you want to improve family nutrition you need to see what is already available in your locality. Where do families shop? Existing provision, local supermarkets, markets (including fast food outlets), and transport services. Health promotional opportunities need to be real and reflect local needs, find out what families want, have they already made changes, what could you add to this? Are any other agencies already providing input that you could join? Educational and health promotional opportunities may require a more proactive stance.

Summary

The reality of health visiting practice: public health in the twenty-first century

Health inequalities exist and remain part of the fabric of our society [90]. Despite government rhetoric and policies influencing public health practice, inequalities cannot be solved by simply improving or redirecting health care provision. Factors such as poor or inadequate housing, unemployment, low wages and deprivation contribute to inequalities requiring policies to address them. Health is political and must be viewed as such if inequality, inequity and disparity are truly to be addressed. Health visitors need to be mindful of this and their valuable contribution.

The Darzi Report [30] discusses improved services and focuses on quality and health care, choices and partnership working. All of these attributes are commendable; however, if the minimum wage does not rise and investment in social housing remains protracted then individuals and families will not feel valued and this will inevitably lead to further inequalities whereby, families and communities will become marginalised. In addition, families, individuals and communities will become less inclined to participate actively in their health choices. Health visitors need to be politically astute, and view health potential from a broader perspective which will facilitate and enable change from within the community, turning government rhetoric into reality.

The full disclosure: health visiting facts

What health visitors need to do to address inequalities in health

- Assess need in your community (apply the concept of need and build a profile) [104]
- Target inequality and inequity within your community (provide opportunities for hidden and minority groups) [105]
- Engage and involve the community in their health care (build social capital)
- Work collaboratively (including intersectoral working)
- Evaluate and justify actions/decisions (knowledge from research) [106]
- Publish findings [107]
- Share practice (all outcomes are not necessarily favourable, nevertheless this is a learning opportunity)
- Consolidate your knowledge of community public health continually (get involved in shared learning opportunities) [108]
- **Remember: The health visitor's public health potential has yet to be realised** [14].

References

1 Robotham A, Sheldrake D. *Health Visiting: Specialist and Higher Level Practice*. London: Churchill Livingstone, 2000.
2 Robotham A, Frost M. *Health Visiting: Specialist Community Public Health Nursing*, 2nd edn. London: Churchill Livingstone, 2005.
3 Dingwall R. Collectivism, regionalism and feminism: health visiting and British Social Policy 1850-1975. *Journal of Social Policy* 1977; **6**(3): 291-315.
4 Cunningham P. *The Principles of Health Visiting*. London: Faber and Faber Limited, 1967.
5 Ashton J, Seymour H. *The New Public Health*. Milton Keynes: Open University Press, 1988.
6 Aveson J. Biblewomen and sanitary ladies. *Health Visitor* 1987; **60**: 156-61.
7 Douglas J, Earle S, Handsley S, Lloyd C, Spurr S. *A Reader in Promoting Public Health: Challenge and Controversy*. Milton Keynes: Open University Press, and London: Sage, 2007.
8 Clarke J. *A Family Visitor*. London: Royal College of Nursing, 1973.
9 White R. Health visitors: the willing horses. *Health Visitor* 1987; **60**: 163-8.
10 Ministry of Health. *An Inquiry into Health Visiting*. London: HMSO, 1956.
11 Council for the Education and Training of Health Visitors (CETHV). *An Investigation into the Principles of Health Visiting*. London: CETHV, 1977.
12 Council for the Education and Training of Health Visitors (CETHV). *The Investigation Debate: A Commentary on 'An Investigation into the Principles of Health Visiting'*. London: CETHV, 1980.
13 Council for the Education and Training of Health Visitors (CETHV). *Principles in Practice*. London: CETHV, 1982.

14 Cowley S, Frost M. *The Principles of Health Visiting: Opening the Door to Public Health Practice in the 21st century.* London: CPHVA, 2006.

15 Twinn S, Cowley S. *The Principles of Health Visiting: A Re-examination.* London: HVA/UKSC, 1992.

16 Twinn S. Conflicting paradigms of health visiting: a continuing debate for professional practice. *Journal of Advanced Nursing* 1991; **16**: 966-73.

17 Orr J. *Health Visiting in Focus.* London: Royal College of Nursing, 1980.

18 Robinson J. *An Evaluation of Health Visiting.* London: CETHV, 1982.

19 Batley N. *The History of the Council for the Education and Training of Health Visitors: The Middle Years.* London: ENB, 1983.

20 United Kingdom Central Council for Nursing Midwifery and Health Visiting (UKCC). *The Future of Professional Practice.* London: UKCC, 1994.

21 Luker K, Orr J. *Health Visiting: Towards Community Health Nursing.* Oxford: Blackwell Scientific Publications, 1992.

22 Department of Health. *Facing the Future: A Review of the Role of Health Visitors.* London: HMSO, 2007.

23 Department of Health. *The Government Response to Facing the Future.* London: HMSO, 2007.

24 Acheson D (Chair). *An Independent Inquiry into Inequalities in Health.* London: The Stationery Office, 1998.

25 Department of Health. Facing the future: a review of the role of health visitors (available at www.dh.gov.uk/cno); 2007.

26 Department of Health. The government response to facing the future: a review of the role of health visitors (available at http://www.dh.gov.uk/publications); 2007.

27 Goodwin S. *Whiter health visiting? Health Visitor* 1988; **61**(12): 22-5.

28 Brocklehurst N. The new health visiting: thriving at the edge of chaos. *Community Practitioner* 2004; **77**(4): 135-9.

29 Cowley S. *Public Health in Policy and Practice: A Sourcebook for Health Visitors and Community Nurses.* Edinburgh: Bailliere Tindall, 2002.

30 Department of Health. *High Quality Care for All: Next Stage Review Final Report* (Darzi Report). London: HMSO, 2008.

31 Brocklehurst N. Is health visiting 'fully engaged' in its own future well-being? *Community Practitioner* 2004; **77**(6): 214-18.

32 Carr S, Unwin N, Pless-Mulloli T. *An Introduction to Public Health and Epidemiology,* 2nd edn. Maidenhead: Open University Press, 2007.

33 Macdowall W, Bonell C, Davies M. *Health Promotion Practice: Understanding Public Health.* Maidenhead: Open University Press, 2006.

34 Scriven A, Garman S. *Public Health: Social Context and Action.* Maidenhead: Open University Press, 2007.

35 Pencheon D, Guest C, Melzer D, Muir Gray J. *Oxford Handbook of Public Health Practice,* 2nd edn. Oxford: Oxford University Press, 2006.

36 Tones K, Green J. *Health Promotion: Planning and Strategies.* London: Sage, 2004.

37 Corcoran N. *Communicating Health: Strategies for Health Promotion.* London: Sage, 2007.

38 Ewles L. *Key Topics in Public Health: Essential Briefings on Prevention and Health Promotion.* London: Elsevier Churchill Livingstone, 2005.

39 Department of Health. Children's health, our future: a review of progress against the National Service Framework for Children, Young People and Maternity Services 2004 (available at www.dh.gov.uk/publications); 2007.

40 Hall D, Elliman D. *Health for All Children*, 4th edn. Oxford: Oxford University Press, 2003.

41 Department of Health. The Child Health Promotion Programme: Pregnancy and the first five years of life (available at www.dh.gov.uk/publications); 2008.

42 Skidmore D. *The Ideology of Community Care*. London: Chapman & Hall, 1994.

43 Putnam R. *Bowling Alone: The Collapse and Revival of American Community*. New York: Simon & Schuster, 2000.

44 Fitzpatrick T. *Welfare Theory: An Introduction*. Basingstoke: Palgrave, 2001.

45 Blaxter M. How health is experienced? In: Douglas J, Earle S, Handsley S, Lloyd C, Spurr S, eds. *A Reader in Promoting Public Health: Challenge and Controversy*. Milton Keynes: Open University Press, and London: Sage, pp. 19-32, 2007.

46 Laverack G. *Health Promotion Practice: Building Empowered Communities*. Maidenhead: Open University Press, 2007.

47 Labonte R. Health promotion and empowerment: reflections on professional practice. *Health Education Quarterly* 1994; **21**(2): 253-68.

48 Davies M, Macdowell W. *Health Promotion Theory: Understanding Public Health*. Maidenhead: Open University Press, 2006.

49 Gillam S, Yates J, Badrinath P. *Essential Public Health: Theory and Practice*. Cambridge: Cambridge University Press, 2007.

50 Department of Health. *Choosing Health: Making Healthier Choices Easier*. London: HMSO, 2004.

51 Department of Health. *Our Health, Our Care, Our Say: A New Direction for Community Services*. London: HMSO, 2006.

52 Chalmers K. Searching for health needs: the work of health visiting, *Journal of Advanced Nursing* 1993; **18**: 900-11.

53 Maslow A. *Motivation and Personality*. New York: Harper, 1954.

54 Bradshaw J. 'The concept of social need'. *New Society*, 30 March, 1972.

55 Hooper J. Health needs assessment: helping change happen. *Community Practitioner* 1999; **72**(9): 286-8.

56 Dahlgren G, Whitehead M. *Policies and Strategies to Promote Social Equity in Health*. Stockholm: Institute for Futures Studies, 1991.

57 Bayer R, Gostin L, Jennings B, Steinbock B. *Public Health Ethics: Theory, Policy and Practice*. Oxford: Oxford University Press, 2007.

58 Orme J, Powell J, Taylor P, Harrison T, Grey M. *Public Health for the 21st Century: New Perspectives on Policy, Participation and Practice*. Maidenhead: Open University Press, 2003.

59 Power R, French R, Connelly J, George S, Hawes D, Hinton T et al. Health, health promotion and homelessness. *BMJ* 1999; **318**: 590-92.

60 World Health Organization. *Ottawa Charter for Health Promotion*. First International Conference on Health Promotion, Ottawa 17-21 November. Copenhagen: WHO Regional Office for Europe, 1986.

61 World Health Organization. *The Bangkok Charter for Health Promotion in a Globalized World*. 6th Global Conference on Health Promotion. Bangkok: WHO, 2005.

62 Housten A, Cowley S. An empowerment approach to needs assessment in health visiting practice. *Journal of Clinical Nursing* 2002; **11**: 640-50.

63 Whitehead D. Health promotion and health education: advancing the concepts. *Journal of Advanced Nursing* 2004; **47**(3): 311-20.

64 Tones K, Tilford S. *Health Promotion: Effectiveness, Efficiency and Equity*, 3rd edn. Cheltenham: Chapman & Hall, 2001.

65 Smith S, Sinclair D, Raine R, Reeves B. *Health Care Evaluation: Understanding Public Health*. Maidenhead: Open University Press, 2005.

66 Department of Health. *The Health Visitor and School Nurse Development Programme: Health Visitor Practice Development Resource Pack* (available at http://www.innovate.hda.online.org.uk). London: Department of Health, 2001.

67 Almond P. An analysis of the concept of equity and its application to health visiting. *Journal of Advanced Nursing* 2002; **37**(6): 598-606.

68 Burns S, Bulman C. *Reflective Practice in Nursing: The Growth of the Professional Practitioner*, 2nd edn. Oxford: Blackwell Science Limited, 2000.

69 Moon J. *Reflection in Learning & Professional Development: Theory & Practice*. London: Kogan Page Limited, 1999.

70 Kember D et al. *Reflective Teaching & Learning in the Health Professionals*. Oxford: Blackwell Science, 2001.

71 Johns C. *Becoming a Reflective Practitioner*, 2nd edn. Oxford: Blackwell Publishing Limited, 2004.

72 Nursing and Midwifery Council. *Standards to Support Learning and Assessment in Practice*. London: NMC, 2008.

73 Smith M. Health visiting: the public health role. *Journal of Advanced Nursing* 2004; **45**(1): 17-25.

74 Rissell C. Empowerment: the holy grail of health promotion? *Health Promotion International* 1994; **9**(1): 39-47.

75 Kendall S. *Health and Empowerment: Research and Practice*. London: Arnold Publishers, 1998.

76 Gibson C. A concept analysis of empowerment. *Journal of Advanced Nursing* 1991; **16**: 354-61.

77 Wallerstein N, Bernstein E. Empowerment education: Friere's ideas adapted to health education. *Health Education Quarterly* 1988; **15**(4): 379-94.

78 Wallerstein N. Powerlessness, empowerment and health: implications for health promotion programmes. *American Journal of Health Promotion* 1992; **6**(3): 197-205.

79 Wallerstein N. *What Is the Evidence on Effectiveness of Empowerment to Improve Health?* Copenhagen: WHO regional Office for Europe, 2006.

80 Nutbeam D, Harris E. *Theory in a Nutshell: A Practical Guide to Health Promotion Theories*, 2nd edn. Sydney: McGraw-Hill, 2004.

81 Prochaska J, DiClimente C. The transtheoretical (stages of change) model. In: Nutbeam D, Harris E, eds. *Theory in a Nutshell: A Practical Guide to Health Promotion Theories*, 2nd edn. Sydney: McGraw-Hill, 1984.

82 Becker MH, ed. The health belief model and personal health behavior. *Health Education Monography* 1974; **2**: 324-473.

83 Ajzen L, Fishbein M. *Understanding Attitudes and Predicting Social Behavior*. Englewood Cliffs, NJ: Prentice Hall, 1980.

84 Bandura A. *Social Foundations of Thoughts and Actions: A Social Cognitive Theory*. Englewood Cliffs, NJ: Prentice Hall, 1986.

85 Rycroft-Malone J, Seers K, Tichen A, Harvey G, Kitson A, McCormack B. What counts as evidence in evidenced based practice? *Journal of Advanced Nursing* 2004; **47**(1): 81-90.

86 Cooper H, Arber S, Fee L, Ginn J. *The Influence of Social Support and Social Capital on Health: A Review and Analysis of British Data*. London: Health Education Authority, 1999.

87 Morgan A, Popay J. Community participation for health: reducing health inequalities and building social capital. In: Scriven A, Garmen S, eds. *Public Health: Social Context and Action*. Maidenhead: Open University Health, 2007.

88 Campbell C, Wood R, Kelly M. *Social Capital for Health*. London: Health Education Authority, 1999.

89 Gibson A. Does social capital have a role to play in the health of communities? In: Douglas J, Earle S, Handsley S, Lloyd C, Spurr S, eds. *A Reader in Promoting Public Health: Challenge and Controversy*. Milton Keynes: Open University Press, and London: Sage, 2007.

90 Graham H. *Unequal Lives: Health and Socioeconomic Inequalities*. Maidenhead: Open University Press, 2007.

91 Naidoo J, Wills J. *Public Health and Health Promotion: Developing Practice*, 2nd edn. London: Bailliere Tindall, 2005.

92 Alcock P. *Understanding Poverty*, 3rd edn. London: Palgrave Macmillan, 2006.

93 Graham H. Poverty and health: global and national patterns. In: Douglas J, Earle S, Handsley S, Lloyd C, Spurr S, eds. *A Reader in Promoting Public Health: Challenge and Controversy*. Milton Keynes: Open University Press, and London: Sage, 2007.

94 World Health Organization. *Preventing Child Maltreatment: A Guide to Taking Action and Generating Evidence*. Geneva: WHO, 2006.

95 Blakemore K, Griggs E. *Social Policy: An Introduction*, 3rd edn. Maidenhead: Open University Press, 2007.

96 Wanless D. *Securing Good Health for the Whole Population. Final Report*. London: HM Treasury and Department of Health, 2004.

97 Corby B. Child protection work. In: *Child Abuse: Towards a Knowledge Base*. Maidenhead: Open University Press, 2006, pp. 238–45.

98 Gidley B. Sure start: an upstream approach to reducing health inequalities. In: Scriven A, Garmen S, eds. *Public Health: Social Context and Action*. Maidenhead: Open University Health, 2007.

99 Nutbeam D, Bauman A. *Evaluation in a Nutshell: A Practical Guide to the Evaluation of Health Promotional Programmes*. Sydney: McGraw-Hill, 2006.

100 Reynolds M, Blackstock P. A public health approach for preventing child sexual abuse. *Community Practitioner* 2007; **80**(2): 14-15.

101 Department of Health. *National Service Framework for Children, Young People and Maternity Services*. London: HMSO, 2004.

102 Department for Education and Skills. *Every Child Matters: Change for Children*. London: HMSO, 2004.

103 Department of Health. *Saving Lives: Our Healthier Nation*. London: The Stationery Office, 1999.

104 Cowley S, Houston A. A structured health needs assessment tool: acceptability and effectiveness for health visiting. *Journal of Advanced Nursing* 2003; **43**(1): 82-92.

105 Corcoran N, Garlick J. Evidenced-based practice and communication. In: Corcoran N, ed. *Communicating Health: Strategies for Health Promotion*. London: Sage, 2007.

106 Bryans A. Examining health visiting expertise: combining simulation, interview and observation. *Journal of Advanced Nursing* 2004; **47**(6): 623-30.

107 Hillier D, Caan W, McVicar A. Research training and leadership for midwives and health visitors. *Community Practitioner* 2007; **80**(1): 28-33.

108 Grant R. 'Micro' public health – the reality. *Community Practitioner* 2005; **78**(5): 178-82.

Chapter 4
Health Visiting in Practice

Faith Muir and Paul Reynolds

Learning objectives

After reading this chapter you will be able to:

- Define health visiting in a public health context
- Identify the issues that have eroded the public health role of the health visitor in the past
- Appreciate the meaning of life script and the importance of early intervention in improving individual and community life
- Discuss the advantages of community development and recognise the barriers that deter health visitor facilitating such projects
- Appreciate the importance of motivation, both individual and group

---

Introduction

Health visitors (HVs) have a family- and child-centred public health role and deliver this service as part of a wider public health service. Health visiting aims to provide universal early intervention, prevention and health promotion programmes delivered on a continuum of support to all children, young people and families according to need. The profession is required to work in both partnership and collaboration with a variety of agencies and professionals in an innovative and dynamic way that is responsive to children's and families' needs and to tackle public health priorities. It is a progressive universal service which delivers a systematic planned continuum of care and support according to need at a neighbourhood and an individual level, in order to achieve greater equity of outcomes for all children and families. Those with the greatest risks and needs will receive more intensive support from the health visiting service [1].

Health visiting practice is underpinned by the still relevant four principles of health visiting that guide and inform professional practice [2]. These are:

- The search for health needs
- Stimulation of an awareness of health needs

- The influence on policies affecting health
- The facilitation of health-enhancing activities

The Nursing and Midwifery Council (NMC) state within the proficiencies required for Specialist Community Public Health Nursing, that public health is still integral to the role of health visiting and draws our attention to the vulnerable populations within society which are in need of the service.

Public health operates at the 'pre-need' stage, by identifying and fulfilling self-declared and recognised, as well as unrecognised, health needs of individuals and social groups. Paying particular attention to disadvantaged or vulnerable populations, health inequalities and factors that contribute to health and well being in the context of people's lives [3].

The term *public health* is a commonly used expression by health professionals, non-health professionals and politicians and simply speaking it is the promotion of the health of the public. However, it does depend on numerous factors, most of which are the remit of government, i.e. housing, environment, transport and food standards (see Chapters 1 and 2). It is, therefore, a much wider matter than just medical interventions and services as is often cited by the media. Public health, in its widest context, can be characterised by several factors [4]. These are:

- Concern for the health of the whole population
- Concern for the prevention of illness
- Recognition of the social factors, which contribute to health

Yet, what at first appears a straightforward concept is in reality a complex and broader set of issues, which the practitioner needs to be cognisant of and will be discussed later. It could be stated that the confusion over the components of public health has led to a narrow-minded approach by health professionals leading to a limited and constrained delivery of the public health agenda and that HVs as a profession have been culpable in allowing this to occur.

Health inequalities

Health inequalities and the increasing health divide between social groups within the United Kingdom remain a major focus in all recent public health reports [5-10]. It is now a generation since the groundbreaking Black report [11] concluded that early childhood is a period of life when effective intervention could hopefully weaken the continuing association between health and social class within the United Kingdom. The Acheson report [12] reinforced this notion of the health divide and stated that the best chance of reducing widespread inequalities in mental and physical health relate directly to improving interventions to parents particularly present and future mothers, and their children. He recommended that this could in part be delivered by the health visiting profession and that the role of the HV should be expanded upon to provide social and emotional support to expectant parents and parents with young children. The Wanless report [13] continued the debate and redefined public health for the twenty-first century by incorporating the collective efforts of individuals and their families.

This reappraisal allowed HVs to fully engage in the process of public health within their practice areas and this was reinforced by the launch of the HV resource pack [14], which demonstrated that public health is a continuum which allowed the practitioners to view their work with individuals, communities and populations as part of the same scale and thereby connected as opposed to viewing them as separate matters. As Robotham and Frost [15] state that HVs tend to work within two models of health: the medical and social models. It is this ability to incorporate both models into practice which allows the HV to offer a public health perspective which focuses on the prevention of illness and disease and the promotion of health whilst acknowledging the contributing factors of social, economic and environmental determinants of health.

Health visitor's role

Yet, it is apparent that the public health role of the HV in many areas across the country since the turn of the century has been slowly eroded. The reasons are varied and complex but the general consensus for this decline is that:

- The whole time equivalent of HV hours in many trusts has been reduced with the resultant public health issues being seen as a lesser priority by an overstretched workforce.
- The role of the HV in practice becoming blurred and losing its focus within newly formed primary care organisations, with the profession itself losing sight of its core principles and being pulled towards the medical model at the cost of the social model.
- A devaluation of the clinical leader's role that traditionally has driven practice.
- A lack of understanding of the HV's role and the importance that early intervention can have when dealing with public health matters.
- The role of the HV impinged upon by other professionals and workers both statutory and non-statutory, whose own roles have developed considerably over the last few years. The HV is now part of a larger multi-skilled team in the community and this has taken time to fully acknowledge the complexities of other roles and the implications this has upon the HV's role. Whilst the growth has been broadly welcomed, it nevertheless has caused a period of unsettlement within the profession.
- A poor research base within the profession from which to base its public health activities.

- The pressures on HVs to provide evidence of their activities has led the practice to become a 'number crunching' exercise. In other words, quantity over quality has become the norm in many trusts.

It was, therefore, apposite that the review of the role of the HV [1] occurred whereby the profession was forced to refocus its function within a public health context and to clarify to itself as well as others, its place within the NHS structure. Society has altered considerably over the past few decades with key public health priorities now taking centre stage of any government strategy. One only has to look at the areas HVs are being charged to play a lead role upon to realise the enormity of the public health agenda. To name a few:

- Social exclusion in children and families
- Obesity
- Smoking cessation
- Child and family mental health
- Drug and alcohol misuse
- Accident prevention

Within the children, young people and families' public health service, the re-mit of the HV is primarily to focus on early intervention, prevention and health promotion of children and their families through a public health approach. The HV will lead the Child Health Promotion Programme (CHPP) [16] whilst maintaining a hand on role. This will require those practitioners with highly developed complex skills to continue in the role they are good at and not be drawn away from the child and family. The profession will:

- Lead and deliver in partnership with other agencies and professionals in a range of settings through a public health approach, the universal CHPP
- Lead and deliver wider community public health packages related to the health and well-being of young children and their families
- Deliver intensive therapeutic programmes to the most disadvantaged young children and families

The stage is now set for the profession to refocus its attentions onto the varied public health issues, which currently affect individuals, communities and population as a whole.

Targets for health

It must be accepted that targets are a part of the NHS and within the public health domain it is no different. The public sector agreement [10] target is that, by 2010, to reduce inequalities in health outcomes by 10% as measured by infant mortality and life expectancy at birth. This is underpinned by the objective on reducing infant mortality and by starting with children, under one year, by 2010 to reduce by at least 10% the gap in mortality between the routine and manual group and the population as a whole. The government views the reductions in infant mortality as a key marker in its attempts to reduce the widening health divide.

Influencing child health

Early childhood development is defined as the period from prenatal to eight years of age and has been recognised by policy makers as a key social determinant of health and health inequalities [17]. Cowley et al. [18] acknowledge that this is the age, which HVs have predominately focused upon, and that the profession still uses this base to reach out to the wider community in which children and their families live in order to influence the structural determinants of health. It is, therefore, obvious that the health visiting profession is still central to any sustainable public health agenda, which concentrates on the welfare of children and their families.

Investment in early childhood is the most effective investment a country can make, with returns over the lifetime many times the size of the original investment. What a child experiences during its early years will set a critical foundation for its entire life course [17]. The term *life script* is becoming commonplace and essentially this entails recognising that we all have a life story, which will take us through to end or the final curtain. For some this script is smooth and full of opportunity, whilst for others it is fraught with traumas and a distinct lack of opportunity. The role of the professional is to understand the potential life story of their client within their community and to empower the transformation from a negative script to a positive script.

From a childhood perspective those first few years are vital and their importance cannot be underestimated. The three broad domains of development whether physical, social or cognitive are interconnected and are equally important for the child. Social determinants shape brain and biological development through their influence on the qualities of stimulation and nurturance.

Inequalities in health can be significantly reduced by the instigation of breastfeeding and the later introduction of solids [19]. This study concluded that home visiting by effective HVs led to an array of health improvements in the child and family. These were:

- Increased breastfeeding rates
- Amelioration of behavioural problems including sleep
- Reduction in non-accidental injuries
- Increased parenting skills
- Increased intellectual abilities in children

It must be reiterated that the term highlighted above is 'effective'. There is little point in health visiting unless the practitioner is able to make a difference in the family or the community in which she serves. It is not a question of just visiting or 'popping in' but to behave in a systematic, planned manner providing therapeutic interventions and evidence-based practice.

The government has as one of its core manifesto aims to redress the disadvantages of being born into a particular social class has on the individual. It is a sobering reminder that the association between growing up in poverty and being poor in adulthood has strengthened since the 1970s. There is little doubt that poverty damages children and it is surmised that by three years of age, poverty makes a difference equivalent to nine months' developmental delay. By 14 years of age the delay is nearly for 2 years. Indeed, the greater the number of risks children face (internal and external), the greater will be their vulnerability to poorer health, developmental delay and psychological difficulties [20]. Evidence suggests that simply being born into a different social class will have a significant effect on the life expectancy of that individual. The life expectancy of a male in Glasgow city is 11 years less than for the man in East Dorset [21]. It may seem difficult to acknowledge that this health divide continues within the United Kingdom and to feel that the poor are somewhat to blame for their own predicament. However, it is worth remembering that the non-poor in virtually every country blame the poor for their own condition, thereby freeing themselves of any guilt or social obligation [22].

As with most public health matters, change often takes a generation to filter through but government policy has aggressively tackled some of the major contributing factors to health inequality, either directly such as the public smoking ban or indirectly such as the introduction of the minimum wage.

Whether some of these initiatives have been successful or not is debatable and will often depend upon political perspectives. However, it has ensured that the nation's health is under constant scrutiny and that all health professionals are charged to implement change. It is worth noting that HVs need to be politically astute in their practice to understand the health and social policy drivers being implemented and to be cognisant of its repercussions. Without understanding the basics of government policy and how it relates to local populations, the HV could be accused of disadvantaging the community and failing to address one of the principles of practice, namely, to influence policies affecting health.

The continual reinforcement of the cycle of poverty occurs because children learn poverty-induced values and attitudes from their parents. Therefore, they learn a set of beliefs, which include apathy, resignation, fatalism, immediate gratification, early sexual encounters and a mistrust of authority [23]. This learnt behaviour is challenging to overcome for all professionals as often these values are in direct opposition to our own and we feel that we just scratching the surface of the problem. It is notable that research coming through from the Sure Start areas is pointing towards highly skilled practitioners delivering the best outcomes for that community and that the family health partnership pilot projects in various Primary Health Care Trusts are concentrating on delivering intensive packages of therapeutic input to targeted families from the antenatal period to when the child is two years of age.

Stable employment of parents and sound education are the two most important routes out of poverty for children [24]. It is vital that the HV recognises her connectivity to both education and employment matters locally and nationally and to explore those opportunities to work collaboratively within her locality. This again supports the argument for early therapeutic interventions that increase the chances of children reaching their potential and increasing parental confidence that gives communities a better chance to access work and education. The HV needs to be aware of the 'bigger picture' if she is to be a true advocate for her community in which she works. The new practitioner has to have a sound awareness of:

- Social exclusion
- Social capital
- Community development
- Vulnerability

These terms are now central to practice for HVs and should inform and guide practice.

Social exclusion

Social exclusion is what can happen when individuals suffer from a combination of linked problems such as unemployment, poor skills, low incomes, poor housing, high crime environments, bad health and family breakdown [25]. Yet, social exclusion also refers to factors resulting in people being excluded from normal exchanges, practices and rights of modern society. Poverty is one of the most obvious factors but social exclusion also refers to inadequate rights in housing, education, health and access to services. A two-tier society is becoming evident [26].

Dimensions of social exclusion which the HV needs to be aware of are:

- Economic: This takes into account factors relating to unemployment, job insecurity, workless homes and income poverty.
- Social: Refers to the possible breakdown of relationships, teenage pregnancies, disaffected youths and crime.
- Neighbourhood: Decaying housing stock, collapse of social networks and withdrawal of services from the most deprived areas because of vandalism and fears for staff safety.
- Political: Feelings of disempowerment, voter apathy with poor electoral turnout and social disturbance.
- Individual: Clients with mental and physical conditions and educationally low achievers are more likely to find themselves socially excluded.
- Spatial: Refers to the concentration of vulnerable groups in often quite distinct areas resulting in whole wraiths of cities and towns becoming economic wastelands.
- Group: Refers to the concentration of the above characteristics in particular groups, i.e. elderly, disabled and ethnic minorities.

When faced with a community of deprivation, the HV may feel overwhelmed by the scale of the problems she encounters. One avenue she should take to gain an accurate snapshot of the issues affecting the community she works is to do a community profile.

> ### Activity 4.1
>
> Think about the community you work in. Can you identify families or groups who are either socially excluded or at risk of becoming socially excluded?
> What are the underlying factors, which have led to this situation?
> In an ideal world what could be done to help?
> What can you do as a health visitor to redress this exclusion?

Community profiling

Profiling represents a traditional health visiting practice that has changed little over the years. It is fair to say that it has fallen out of fashion in recent times due to a number of reasons. Robotham and Sheldrake [27] identify that practice has not been responsive to the identified need of the local population because of two factors. Firstly, the organisational management of the HVs has meant their work has been directed by local policies and management structures which are not sensitive to the smaller communities the practitioner may be working in. The patch covered by the profile may well be quite different to neighbouring communities, i.e. a particularly high incidence of children with special needs or illicit drug-using mothers. Within the realms of the Primary Care Trusts, this may represent a relatively small concern, which may detract from perceived more pressing matters, but within a community it could be a significant public health issue.

Secondly, HVs have found it difficult to work with the increasingly available social data carried out by statutory and non-statutory agencies, which tends to balance need with the resources available such as housing. The HV who essentially works from an illness prevention and health promotion perspective struggles with this type of data.

However, the community profile is, if carried out correctly, a tremendously useful proactive work piece which should guide practice and allows the practitioner to truly know her community. It is a comprehensive description of the community and the health and social needs of that identified community. It should also highlight the available resources both financially and non-financially that exist within the community. It can draw upon both physical and social capital within a 'patch' to highlight key assets for the community. Finally, an action plan can be developed to redress some of the health and social needs of that group of people.

Profiling is a key skill in the HV's toolkit. It allows the practitioner to build up a collection of data which identifies both the health and social needs of the public in which they work. It should not be carried out in isolation, rather the underpinning philosophy of any profile should be the communication and collaboration required between professional groups and more importantly the individuals and groups of the community in question. Information that in an academic sense would be classed as anecdotal can be very useful when building a picture of the community. An individual's and a community's perception of what their environment is like can be very eye-opening.

Activity 4.2

What data could be collected to carry out a community profile in your area of work?
Bear in mind that social and health data is required.
Who would you involve?
Where would you collect the data from and how would you present it?

Social capital

Social capital is a term increasingly used within the health and social arena. Yet, the concept has been around for over a century. Putnam [28] cites Hanifan definition of social capital in 1916 as:

The community as a whole will benefit by the co-operation of all its parts, while the individual will find in his associations, the advantages of the help, the sympathy and the fellowship of his neighbours.

To clarify further, physical capital refers to the buildings and infrastructure of a community, whilst social capital is essentially about the people within that area. It is just as important as the physical capital yet is often overlooked when profiling is carried out. Why is it that some communities have vibrancy about them when you visit them? There always seems to be events occurring, people talking to each other and a general feel good factor. It is not necessarily about money, it is about the people and the individuals who make up that community and make it function. Putnam elaborates by identifying components of social capital as social bridging and social bonding.

Social bridging

The social bridging aspect is essentially inclusive and is outward looking and will encompass people from diverse social backgrounds, i.e. playgroups and schools. Whilst bonding is exclusive and refers to those groups, which by choice or necessity are inward looking, i.e. church groups. Within a community both are important, bridging can generate broader identities whereas bonding can bolster the narrower self. As Putnam states that bonding is good for getting by while bridging is crucial for getting ahead. Bonding is the superglue whilst bridging is the oil that lubricates communities.

Within many communities there has been a breakdown in trust and respect for each other. The reasons are varied and complex but essentially society has altered significantly over the past generation. As a nation, we have become more prosperous. We now have a culture, which is of the individual rather than of society. Wealth has allowed us more freedom to do as we please, i.e. to go abroad on holiday, to go to restaurants or buy a new car or the latest plasma widescreen television with 100 channels to watch.

Yet all this comes at a price, we are more likely to get divorced and live alone. We tend to work longer hours in an area away from our own home. We spend more time travelling and we have fewer close social contacts. Or as Putnam prefers to state 'we are bowling alone'. This expression relates to the fact that he is American and if you remember the old films from the 1950s and 60s, often the lead characters would be seen in groups either going ten-pin bowling or playing cards together at home. Putnam laments the demise of this culture and noticed the correlation between the decline in social events and the decline in society. It is commented upon that large numbers of well-educated middle class young men and women withdrew from clubs and churches, thereby detaching themselves from strong supportive networks. This civic disengagement was passed onto their children and hence the predicament society finds itself in. Interestingly, opting out of religion leaves a major void for individuals which needs filling. As Stephen Fry remarked, 'stop believing in God and the majority of people will believe in everything!'

It is proposed that communities which are high in social capital fare much better than those which are not. By dealing with the smaller things, which affect us, and which we have control over, then the larger problems afflicting the community will be reduced. For example, by taking an interest in the welfare of elderly neighbours or by joining the local school board of governors, then you are actively engaged in that community. Social networks develop and commonalities are forged. Individuals would start taking a pride in their neighbour and keep a watch over events. If these small steps occur then the possibilities are endless. It is surmised that the following would happen:

- Violence reduces
- Teenage pregnancies decline
- Infant mortality rates reduce
- Low-birth-weight babies are fewer
- Poverty reduces
- Obesity rates would decline

The overall philosophy is that as individuals we lack a voice but as a group we start to become empowered, we feel more confident and we are no longer alone. Let us take the obesity issue from the above list. If a parent were on the local school board of governors, he or she would be able to influence decisions about the sporting facilities being utilised out of school hours. Potentially the gymnasium and sports field could be hired out to interested parties or even groups of parents who might want to set up a 5-a-side league, for example. The local HVs could facilitate the setting up of exercise classes. The school with a little effort could become the central focus for the community. Instead of having high fences around the perimeter with signs saying to keep out, it could be transformed into a meeting place. Instead of having schools which are empty for large periods of time and run the risk of being subject to arson attacks, which unfortunately is becoming the norm. The local population see it as theirs and something to cherish and become involved in. The obesity problem is at least tackled from a community perspective.

Networking has long been a highly prized skill that HVs acquire. The HV is ideally placed to introduce families to appropriate groups, from Smoking Cessation Groups, a parenting group to a library parent and baby group. The groups help parents grow in confidence and social capital.

Social capital initiatives often require a degree of lateral thinking from HVs but the opportunities are there to be innovative. Although it can be perceived as being rather simplistic in its concept and some critics have declared that social capital is an attempt to fill the void left by reduced public services. Undoubtedly, social capital is not the answer to all of societies' ills or to all of the public health issues affecting the country but it can be enhanced to limit the damage poverty can inflict on a community. By having repeated interactions with fellow citizens with a neighbourhood, individuals will develop and maintain traits that are good for society. These traits are tolerance, empathy and less cynicism.

Activity 4.3

Think of public health issue affecting the community you work in.
How could you tackle this problem by building social capital?
What would you do?
Who would you approach?

Community development

Running in tandem and even overlapping social capital is the concept of community development. Although the term is probably more familiar to HVs than social capital, there still requires clarification of its meaning. Ross [29] defines it as:

A process by which a community identifies its needs or objectives, ranks these needs or objectives, develops the confidence to work at these needs or objectives, find resources to deal with these needs or objectives, takes action in respect to them, and in so doing extends and develops co-operative and collaborative attitudes and practices in the community.

HVs have often found community development difficult to become truly engaged in, due to managerial policies requiring them to quantify their work in measurable terms. However, from a public health perspective, community development is a vital aspect of the profession, which should be nurtured by managers who need to take a long-term attitude to this type of work. It is also fair to add that the development of Sure Start programmes across the country has impinged upon the role of the HV in this area and that professional rivalries and ideologies have led to some HVs being marginalised. There is evidence to suggest that this is changing and the health input and knowledge HVs have of a specific geographic area is of the utmost importance.

Naidoo and Wills [4] suggest that community development is both a philosophy and a method. They cite the following points as central to the concept:

- A commitment to equality
- An emphasis on participation and enabling the community to be heard
- Valuing people's own experiences
- Collecting experiences and seeing problems as shared
- Empowering individuals and communities through education, skills development and joint action

There needs to be an underlying belief from the HV that the community in which she serves has a fundamental right to achieve its health and social potential. Whilst this stance may appear political in nature, it could be argued that the health visiting profession needs to become more political astute if they are to fully support, facilitate and empower their community. Community development is as much to do with recognising people's rights to equity of services and potential for equality as well as the actual mechanics of the development.

From a HV perspective the link between strong community development and good health seems obvious, yet the initial steps can appear daunting. All community development takes time and this is because the main component is, that it has to be user led. The role of the HV is as a facilitator and catalyst and caution needs to be made to avoid the easy trap of prescribing for the community. In others words it is common mistake for health professionals to take one look at the problems facing a populace and to recommend a course of action to rectify it without truly knowing the individuals or groups involved. This approach will smack of paternalism and will rightly be met with indignation and resentment. Management structures within NHS trusts that require number of contacts and outcomes can often reinforce the HV's reluctance to become involved.

Instead, the HV will need to adopt the following three traits to fully engage in community development. These according to Naidoo and Wills [4] are:

- To be user led and to understand the priorities a community has rather than inflicting external priorities onto them.
- To focus on the process of enablement. By allowing individuals and groups to participate in identifying their own health and social needs will in itself be a positive action. Self-esteem and confidence will be improved and these in themselves are health-promoting factors.

- To concentrate on the vulnerable and disadvantaged groups. Instead of focusing on individual lifestyles and running the risk of stigmatising those individuals. Community development should be concerned with the social determinants of ill health and be aimed at empowering people and groups to act together to influence issues, which affect them. This may be to do with housing, politics, crime, street lighting or even dog fouling. The main thing is that it is about their priorities for addressing their health and social needs.

To summarise, then, HVs need to ask the people what they think about their community and what would make things better and remember their priorities may be quite different from yours.

An example of community development from health visiting practice was the setting up of a postnatal depression group for mothers within a defined area. It had become apparent from conversations with mothers who were experiencing a mental health problem following the birth of their child, on caseloads that there was a need to provide a support group for them. They complained of feeling isolated, guilty and scared; they felt they were the only ones with this problem and expressed a desire to meet up with other women going through the same process. Initially, there had been some concerns raised from professionals and management about:

- Risk management
- Cost
- Time required to organise
- Appropriate venue

However, these were resolved and what commenced rather tentatively with a handful of participants and health professionals including a proactive mid-wife and psychiatric nurse, quickly grew to become a well-established and well-attended postnatal depression group with a range of services aimed for the local populace. The group rapidly moved from the safe medical perspective of explaining depression etc. to a broad social model providing emotional support and practical help. The professionals involved understood this development and though pride might have hurt by the power shift towards the lay community, this had to occur for the group to survive. The group after all was theirs to do as it pleased. The health professionals still maintained a therapeutic input, particularly for new attendees and were still a resource of expert knowledge but the balance had shifted. The mothers themselves:

- Organised a telephone support helpline
- Raised money via a number of charity events, which helped fund crèche facilities and transport
- Appeared on local television to highlight the plight of depressed women in society
- Presented at a conference

- Lobbied the local Primary Care Trust and Social Services for additional funds

What at first seemed like a major task for the health professionals, very quickly turned out to be the most rewarding aspect of their job. The evaluation of the project revealed that the time spent setting up the project was repaid many times over by the success of it. Not only was the HV's time spent on maternal mental health issues reduced but also it was concluded that the GP, midwife and community psychiatric nurses' time was saved as well. The mothers' mental illness was obviously a priority to be addressed by the group but the dynamics of the group itself helped increase the individual's self-esteem, confidence and provide a sense of belonging when they felt adrift in a sea of despair. Whilst the health professionals were trying their best to cope with these women on an individual basis, they could never hope to match what the women could provide for each other. In reality, HVs struggle to provide an hour a week to someone of their caseload who is depressed. Yet a supportive group with befriending facilities from women who have either gone through the experience themselves or were going through it also, could provide a significant amount of time, which the HV could never match.

What must be remembered is that not all projects or community develop-ment will be successful and that is to be expected. What must be allowed, however, is that it is directed by the community and is supported by the HV in collaboration with other professional and agencies.

True collaboration requires the HV to have the following attitudes and ap-titudes [30]:

- Reciprocal approach
- Flexibility
- Integrity

As well as the following skills:

- Open communication
- Relational skills
- Organisational skills
- Helping manner

Barriers to collaboration should be tackled both on an individual level and on an organisational level.

Barriers to communication:

- Professional tribalism
- Spending constraints
- Different accountabilities
- Core beliefs of individuals involved
- Looking at things from one angle

> **Activity 4.4**
>
> Think of the advantages and disadvantages of community development. How could you persuade your line manager that you should be involved in a community development project around road safety issues? What would the health benefits be?

Vulnerability

The concept of vulnerability is commonplace in discussions of adult and child protection and in health and welfare provision more generally. Indeed many services are planned and organised around the provision of services to vulnerable groups. It could be argued that the notion of vulnerability widely permeates contemporary models of health promotion and social inclusion. However, the precise meaning of the term can lead to confusion, as it is not always made clear when an individual or group is deemed vulnerable. At the level of service delivery, risk assessment plays a disproportionate role in the diagnosis of vulnerability. Although risk assessment is clearly important it must be considered in relation to the context and situation before vulnerability is measured. A definition, however, is important and the following from the Department of Health [31] is a useful starting point. Vulnerability is:

> A person who is in need of community care services by reason of mental or other disabilities, age or illness and who is or may be unable to take care of themselves or unable to protect themselves against significant harm or exploitation.

It has been suggested that we are becoming more vulnerable as a society [32] yet what components make up vulnerability? Lessick et al. [33] suggest that our inborn characteristics determine a threshold of vulnerability and this is unique to each individual. If the level of vulnerability remains below the threshold level, the person is able to cope, adapt and remain healthy. Conversely, if the threshold level is exceeded then harm will occur to that person. In other words, vulnerability is a continuum on which we are all placed. Some cope better than others with stressful situations but it is an individual matter. It would be unfair to say that all elderly people in the United Kingdom are vulnerable. Clearly, this is not the case. We know that some are and some are not whilst others move in and out of states of vulnerability.

Aday [34] identified seven determinants of vulnerability in relation to ill health. These include:

- Age
- Gender
- Race and ethnicity
- Social support
- Education

- Life change
- Income

She continues to differentiate between vulnerability states on the basis of whether the danger comes from within or is environmental. Internal refers to the person who is genetically predisposed to illness or who has little motivation. Environmental refers to external factors often beyond the control of the individual, i.e. marital disharmony or homelessness. Yet it is often the case that the vulnerability threshold is breeched by a number of contributing factors coming from within and without. Appleton [35] agrees and in the context of child and adult protection argues that it is rarely one factor, which places a child or adult at risk of harm. However, it is important to note that not all risks are equal and some factors may have a spiralling effect on the child and family.

The notion of interplay is now widely employed and is reproduced within the concept of a risk triangle. The idea being that vulnerability is a function of three interrelated elements. These are:

- Risk factors
- Resources
- Life experiences

Altering any one of these factors can alter the individual's susceptibility to harm and their capacity to recover.

Risk factors
The importance of knowing about risk factors is that they act as the yardstick for prevention. However, referring to an individual or group as vulnerable is meaningless unless we can be precise about their predisposition to harm. Vulnerability is often based on averages and general descriptors of risk such as a lack of social support or being female or being elderly. Whilst theses are starting points to understanding the social problem of abuse or neglect, risk factors in themselves are not absolute predictors of harm. Interestingly, if a vulnerable family does not meet the typical profile of being at risk, then they may be overlooked or their predicament may be discounted in favour of another family who more accurately reflects the victim profile.

Spiers [36] stresses that if vulnerability is defined predominately in terms of deficits, needs and a functional incapacity to protect oneself from harm the protection strategies may lead to:

- Fragmentation of care
- Potential to blame victims for their situation
- Stereotyping

The advantage of viewing vulnerability as a lived experience is that it avoids regarding individuals susceptible to harm as being an inevitable consequence of gender, socioeconomic status or age. Instead, vulnerability can be measured in terms of an individual's self-perception and is an estimate of their coping skills and level of empowerment. This broadens our understanding of vulnerability and leads the health professional to promote an individualistic approach to assessment and also focuses on vulnerability as a dimension of the quality of life.

A narrow view of vulnerability as a series of risk factors promotes a tick box approach to the diagnosis of vulnerability. The effects of being labelled vulnerable can be extremely stigmatising to children, families and individual adults, and act as a form of social control. This labelling can in itself be a disempowering factor to families and the child could become more disadvantaged. It is interesting to note that vulnerable families and hard-to-reach families are less likely to accept health visiting support or intervention unless services are seen as a universal entitlement [37]. Families who fear stigmatisation within the community they reside see this narrow targeting as a policing approach. An alternative and arguably preferable way to address vulnerability is to focus on the experience of vulnerability and to assess strengths and coping capacity rather than deficits and dependency.

The increasing pressure on agencies to use vulnerability as a conceptual paradigm against which needs can be prioritised, should be resisted on the grounds that normative need is contested and vulnerability is variable.

Activity 4.5

Read the following scenario and consider your response as a HV.
Take into account the welfare of the child and examine the options available to you within your role.
You visit a family who has recently moved into the area. On your visit the young single mother of a two-year-old girl reveals to you that she is an illicit drug user. She is, however, on a methadone programme and is being monitored by the drug outreach team from the local hospital. She is finding the programme challenging and is prone to moodswings.
The family moved to your patch to be closer to the maternal grandparents who are taking an active role in the care of the girl. They visit on a daily basis and sometimes the child spends weekends at the grandparent's house to give the mother a break.
There appears to be a sound attachment between the mother and child and the child's development appears to be within the normal range for this age.
The child has no contact with her father.
What are the main factors within this family?
Who do you discuss this situation with?
Is this family vulnerable?
Is the child at significant risk?

Motivation

When working with many families who are deemed vulnerable one of the main challenges facing the HV can be the family's lack of motivation or desire to change potentially health-damaging activities. We have all faced the family whose diet is nutritionally lacking. Or the smokers who knowing the risks to themselves and their children insist on their daily nicotine fix. Or the mother whose child refuses to go to bed and despite your best attempts to instigate a bedtime routine and action plan for when the child gets up finds it impossible to do even one night of this new regime. So what is happening here? Why do we all engage in activities, which we know deep down is harmful to us or is affecting the quality if our life and relationships, but we still fail to deal with it?

Changing behaviour

The shelves at the local library are full of self-help books for those of us wanting to change our lifestyles. But we still fail to follow through on that healthy guidance which is written in black and white. How many times have you said to yourself that once things have settled down you were going to join that gym, go on that diet, take up a new hobby and learn a foreign language? We have all been there and for most of us those good intentions stay as simply that. There have been a variety of models looking at motivation and change. Perhaps one of the most famous has been Prochaska and DiClemente [38] cycle of change model. This is often used in association with smokers to assess whether they are ready to alter their behaviour. Briefly, it is broken down into five stages where the smoker will be. They are:

- **Pre-contemplation:** This is where the smoker is not even thinking about quitting. They are often quite happy smoking and see no reason to alter.
- **Contemplation:** This is where the smoker is just starting to think about changing their behaviour. Something may have triggered this stage which has caused them to think about their actions, i.e. a new relationship or a health scare.
- **Preparation:** This is where behaviour is changing albeit off and on. They will be seeking out information about quitting and seeking out professionals and groups they can utilise.
- **Action:** This is where behaviour has changed consistently for a short period of time, usually for up to six months. They well may be prone to relapse at times of stress.
- **Maintenance:** It is the final stage when any change has been maintained for over six months and the person now views himself or herself as a non-smoker.

Some smokers move quickly through these stages whilst others never shift from the first stage. Yet as a HV how do you motivate individuals generally (not just smokers)?

Motivation can be simplified into people who are ready to change. A highly motivated person is ready to change whilst a poorly motivated person is not ready to alter. As Johnson [39] states the two key components to motivation are:

- Importance
- Confidence

By increasing the importance, to a client of changing behaviour, this can lead to an increase in motivation and by creating more motivation moves the client faster through the stages of change, whereas by increasing confidence that the client can change a behaviour will create more motivation.

The first component relates to those individuals who often have the confidence to change but do not see the importance of it, whilst the second component refers to the majority of people who acknowledge the importance of changing but lack the confidence to carry this through.

This strategy can relate to any health behaviour, such as exercising, smoking or parenting.

The role of the HV often in behavioural change is to understand where the client is in relation to the change model and to work in partnership with them to understand their needs fuller. It is not as simple as to say stop smoking or lose weight, because as we know, often logical reasons to do something will often fail to motivate. The competent practitioner should be able to draw upon her diagnostic and assessment skills to ascertain what would really make something important enough to alter behaviour. Let us imagine the following scenario, which is a fairly common situation of a young mother with a three-year-old child with a disturbed sleep pattern. The mother has called for your advice because she is at the end of her tether. She is tired and tearful and has tried a number of times to correct his sleep pattern. He used to be a good sleeper but since a bout of chickenpox some time ago, he has altered. The family is obviously quite fraught.

The HV can ascertain fairly quickly that the mother is aware of how important it is for the child and the family that the child gets into a regular sleep pattern. It would appear that she has lost confidence in her ability to carry out the sleep programme necessary. The mother believes that she has tried the sleep programme and it just has not worked for her child. The HV's role is to boost her confidence and to support her through this trying process. Great care is needed not to erode the mother's confidence further by making her feel a failure for not being able to carry the process through to its conclusion. This is not necessarily about motivating her about sleep but to motivate her about her parenting, which has taken a knock in confidence. It will take time but she will achieve her goal of a good night's sleep.

In another situation, you are called to see a mother at home. She has had complaints from other parents at mother and toddler group because her little girl is becoming aggressive. She tells you that her child cannot concentrate on anything and tires herself out that much with crying that she sleeps most of the afternoon, she is worried that her child has attention deficit disorder. When you visit and take a history, you discover that the child is staying up very late with her mother and falling asleep on mum's lap, sometimes as late as midnight, the mother cherishes this time as it is the only time the child is calm and loving. In this case the mother has not seen the importance of a regular sleep pattern and therefore the HV needs to work with her to identify something about altering the behaviour, which the mother would see as important, and clearly it would be her worries about the child's behaviour. If the child slept better she could improve her behaviour. This scenario is far more complex than the first case; however, the key to change is still finding that motivation for change. The mother will benefit by implementing a sleep programme when she has a less disruptive child who is calmer and she can enjoy loving moments throughout the day instead of late at night when they are both probably exhausted.

> ### Activity 4.6
>
> You visit a family whose children are on the child protection register for neglect. It has come to your notice that the children have not been taken recently for their speech therapy appointments or immunisations. When questioned, the parents claim that they think the children's speech will improve naturally and children have too many injections now.
> How do you tackle this situation from a motivational aspect?

Assessing need

> ### Activity 4.7
>
> Take a good look at Figure 4.1.
> It is a piece of contemporary art, which is entitled *Home and Garden*.
> What do you see in the painting?
> What do you think it is painted with?
> What does it say to you?
> What do you think influenced the artist's decisions?
> Are your comments influenced by its title?
> What colours do you think the artist used?

Art has been used a lot in the public health arena; however, this is not the purpose for dropping in Figure 4.1. If you are a student it will be useful to ask one of your fellow students what they answered to the questions posed. It will soon become clear that we all look at things differently and the only thing you may agree on is that you are looking at the same image. The shapes may fascinate one of you and how they work with each other and in some cases

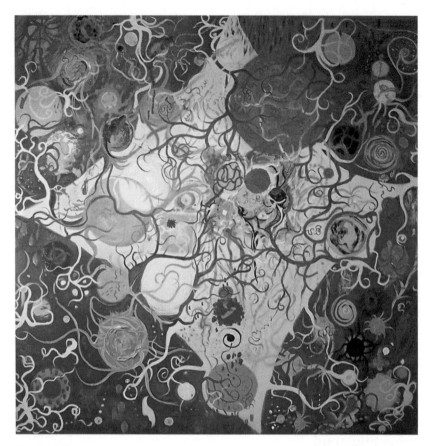

Figure 4.1

oppose each other. One may see chaos and disorder, another may see a busy cheerful painting or you may merely dismiss it as a waste of space. There will be many reasons why each of us sees different things when we look at the painting. We all come from different backgrounds: some come from families who are very creative and have had a childhood surrounded by art and visits to galleries; others will have never set foot in a gallery. Perhaps someone who is reading this has a fine art qualification or is an amateur artist. Whatever your opinion do not take these differences lightly, as it is not just art that individuals see differently and have different opinions about.

When we look at families we see different things. I wager that if you asked ten different professionals what they saw, they would all say something different. Some would focus upon the child and how the child looked and was dressed. Others would look at the family dynamics and the relationships. For example, is the mother close to her child? Is she looking at him or her? Do they seem happy or is that smile fixed and potentially covering something? Others would concentrate on the environment. Do they appear disadvantaged? Is this a family in social decline? There are a myriad of questions, which could be asked, and avenues of thought which could be taken.

It is fair to say that when we assess anything on a snapshot situation like this, then what we are doing is drawing upon years of experience and knowledge sometimes consciously and sometimes subconsciously. We may also be making stereotypical judgements on the families. Who is right? Well, they all are. We all see different things and draw different conclusions but it is important to recognise that as HVs, your opinion is as valid as the next because unlike many other professions, you will have visited or had contact with this family on numerous occasions and have drawn upon a number of assessments to reach your conclusion. Individuals, families and communities are constantly changing and the role of the HV is to facilitate those changes. As in the painting pictured, often what we see initially in a family or a community is confusing, disjointed, and indeed scary but in collaboration with others and the family or community themselves and an open mind an understanding of the issues, which affect this family or the community, will become apparent. It is important to recognise, however, that when we work with other agencies there are two types of models. The first is the developmental model where staff works together for the common good of the client. The second and perhaps most common is the contingency model, which is influenced by workloads, structures and the qualities of staff [40]. Whilst the first model is preferred, it is necessary to understand why the second occurs?

The seven core capabilities for HVs

To be an effective public health practitioner a variety of skills and traits are required.

The seven core capabilities for HVs [41] as outlined in Scotland provide a solid framework from which to practice. They are:

- Assessing the health needs of young children, families and communities: This requires the HV to assess the child's health and developmental needs and to set the child within the context of its family and environment and will include those who are disadvantaged, vulnerable or at risk. There is an expectation that the HV will work in partnership within an integrated team to assess the community needs (profiling) and to develop outcomes to address those needs.
- Promoting health and safeguarding the welfare of the young child: To work in partnership delivering programmes designed to promote health and address key public health issues and inequalities. To ensure that there is an appropriate response to children and families in need of protection from abuse.
- Therapeutic interventions: This will require the HV to provide a range of therapeutic interventions, which will maximise health gain and minimise risk. Evidence-based practice will be central to this concept and would involve independent non-medical prescribing, parenting programmes, behavioural modification, cognitive behavioural therapy, listening visits to name but a few.

- Leadership: There is an expectation that HVs need to lead and facilitate health visiting and children's centre teams to implement policies that takes practice forward. Leadership skills should include seizing opportunities to shape and influence the development of strategies related to improving health and reducing inequalities.
- Integrated working and partnership: Maintaining effective working relationships with families, communities, colleagues and other agencies. Diversity and equality should be the goal respecting race, gender, disability, cultural and sexuality differences.
- Enhancing and developing practice: Continually auditing and evaluating the effectiveness of services for children and families and implementing action plans to support change. There should be a process in place to gain feedback from both stakeholders and clients which would inform and enhance service delivery
- Professional development and learning: The practitioner should be seeking self-improvement through a variety of methods. These could be reflective practice, clinical supervision and individual performance reviews which would link into local and national initiatives.

Whilst this list is not exhaustive it does allow the practitioner to reflect upon there own practice as a HV and provides both the novice and expert worker with a range of skills required to achieve best practice.

Activity 4.8

Spend some time looking at the scenarios below. Try and identify the areas in this chapter that can help you answer the task set. It can be helpful to make some notes.

Scenario 1

It has been brought to your attention that the local infant schools are concerned about the number of overweight children now attending their reception class and have asked you and the school nurse to tackle the problem from a health perspective. You are obviously aware that this is a delicate situation and call a planning meeting with interested agencies to discuss the situation.

Consider a course of action for addressing this issue keeping in mind the roles and skills of other professionals who may be involved in this community.

Scenario 2

The numbers of MMR vaccinations have declined significantly within your patch over the last two years and the PCT are concerned that the low 'herd' immunity levels are placing the local population at risk of developing an outbreak.

How do you approach this matter?

Scenario 3

You work within a relatively deprived area and the breastfeeding rates are disappointingly low. The rates have always been low. What approaches can you as a HV take to begin to increase breastfeeding rates?

Whom will you involve?

Summary

This chapter has covered the fact that the HV has a family- and child-centred public health role and highlighted that investment in early childhood is the most effective investment a country can make. It has also demonstrated that change takes a generation to make an impact but that stable employment of parents and sound education have been shown to be the most important routes out of poverty for children. It has covered the various dimensions of social exclusion, community profiling and that HVs getting involved with communities helps the community develop empowerment. HVs need to be open and work in collaboration with others to be effective, they must assess health needs in order to promote health and facilitate therapeutic interventions. This required leadership qualities combined with professional development.

References

1 Department of Health. *Facing the Future: A Review of the Role of Health Visitors*. London: Department of Health, 2007.

2 Cowley S, Frost M. *The Principles of Health Visiting: Opening the Door to Public Health Practice*. London: CPHVA/UKSC, 2006.

3 Nursing and Midwifery Council. *Standards of Proficiency for Specialist Community Public Health Nursing*. London: NMC, 2004.

4 Naidoo J, Wills J. *Health Promotion: Foundations for Practice*, 2nd edn. Edinburgh: Bailliere Tindall, 2000.

5 Wanless D. *Securing Our Future Health: Taking a Long Term View*. London: HM Treasury, 2002.

6 Department of Health. *Tackling Health Inequalities: A Programme for Action.* London: Department of Health, 2003.

7 Department for Work and Pensions. *Working for Children.* London: The Stationery Office, 2007.

8 Health Inequalities Unit. *Tackling Health Inequalities: 2007 Status Report on the Programme for Action.* London: Health Inequalities Unit, 2008.

9 Department of Health. *Choosing Health: Making Healthy Choices Easier.* London: The Stationery Office, 2004.

10 Department of Health. *Review of the Health Inequalities Infant Mortality PSA Target.* London: Department of Health, 2007.

11 Black D. *Inequalities in Health: Report of a Research Working Group.* London: Department of Health, 1980.

12 Acheson D. *Report of the Independent Inquiry into Inequalities in Health.* London: The Stationery Office, 1998.

13 Wanless D. *Securing Good Health for the Whole Population: Final Report.* London: HM Treasury, 2004.

14 Department of Health. *Health Visitor Practice Development Resource Pack.* London: HMSO, 2001.

15 Robotham A, Frost M. *Health Visiting: Specialist Community Public Health Nursing,* 2nd edn. Edinburgh: Elsevier Churchill Livingstone, 2005.

16 Department for Children, Schools and Families. Department of Health. *The Child Health Promotion Programme. Pregnancy and the First Five Years of Life.* London: Department of Health, 2008.

17 Irwin L, Siddiqi A, Hertzman C. *Early Child Development: A Powerful Equalizer.* Final report for the WHO commission on the social determinants of health. Geneva: World Health Organization, 2007.

18 Cowley S, Cann W, Dowling S, Weir H. What do health visitors do? A national survey of activities and service organisation. *Public Health* 2007; **121**(11): 869-79.

19 Elkan R, Kendrick D, Hewitt M, Robinson JJA, Tolley K, Blair M, et al. The effectiveness of domiciliary health visiting: a systematic review of international studies and a selective review of British literature. *Health Technology Assessment* 2000; **4**(13): 1-339.

20 Montgomery H, Burr R, Woodhead M. *Changing Childhoods.* Maidenhead: Open University Press, 2003.

21 Shaw M, Smith G, Dorling D. Health inequalities and new labour: how the promises compare with real progress. *BMJ* 2005; **330**:1016-21.

22 Gans H. *War Against the Poor.* New York: Basic Books, 1995.

23 Parrillo V. *Contemporary Social Problems,* 5th edn. Boston: Allyn & Bacon, 2002.

24 Blanden J, Gibbons S, for Joseph Rowntree Foundation. *The Persistence of Poverty Across Generations: A View from Two British Cohorts.* Bristol: The Policy Press, 2006.

25 Social Exclusion Unit. *Social Exclusion Unit: Purpose, Work Priorities and Working Methods.* London: HMSO, 1997.

26 Percy-Smith J. *Policy Responses to Social Exclusion: Towards Inclusion?* Maidenhead: Open University Press, 2002.

27 Robotham A, Sheldrake D. *Health Visiting: Specialist and Higher Level Practice.* Edinburgh: Churchill Livingstone, 2000.

28 Putnam R. *Bowling Alone: The Collapse and Revival of American Community.* New York: Simon & Schuster, 2001.

29 Ross M. *Community Organisations: Theories and Principles.* New York: Harper and Brothers, 1955.

30 Hornby S, Atkins J. *Collaborative Care: Inter Professional, Interagency, Interpersonal.* London: Blackwell Scientific, 2000.

31 Department of Health. *No Secrets: Guidance on Developing and Implementing Multi-Agency Policies and Procedures to Protect Vulnerable Adults from Abuse.* London: Department of Health, 2000.

32 Rogers A. Vulnerability, health and healthcare. *Journal of Advanced Nursing* 1997; **26**(1): 65–72.

33 Lessick M, Woodring BC, Naber S, Halstead L. Vulnerability: a conceptual model applied to perinatal and neonatal nursing. *Journal of Perinatal Neonatal Nursing* 1992; **6**(3): 1–14.

34 Aday L. Health status of vulnerable populations. *Annual Review of Public Health* 1994; **15**: 487–509.

35 Appleton J. Working with vulnerable families: a health visitor's perspective. *Journal of Advanced Nursing* 1996; **23**(5): 912–18.

36 Spiers J. New perspectives in vulnerability using emic and etic approaches. *Journal of Advanced Nursing* 2000; **31**(3): 715–21.

37 Apps J, Reynolds J, Ashby V, Husain F. *Family Support in Sure Start Children's Centres: Planning, Commissioning and Delivering.* London: Family and Parenting Institute, 2007.

38 Prochaska JO, DiClemente CC, Norcross JC. In search of how people change. *American Psychologist* 1992; **47**: 1102–14.

39 Johnson J. *The Sixty Second Motivator.* Indianapolis: Dog Ear Publishing, 2006.

40 Payne M. *Social Work and Community Care.* London: Macmillan, 1995.

41 NHS Education for Scotland. *Supporting the Development of Advanced Nursing Practice. A Toolkit Approach.* Edinburgh: CNO Directorate, Scottish Government, 2008.

Chapter 5

The Development of School Nursing

Mary Smith and Sarah Sherwin

Learning objectives

After reading this chapter you will be able to:

- Appreciate the historical, political, legal and social influences affecting the development of the school health services and school nursing
- Discuss the development of legal accountability for school nurses
- Appreciate the standards required of school nurses when promoting the health of the school-aged population

Introduction

This chapter will discuss the historical development of the school health service from its origins in the 1870s and include an exploration of how the public health nursing role of the school nurse has evolved to what it is today in the twenty-first-century United Kingdom (UK). The relevant drivers for public health change, legislation and social policy will be considered in order to appreciate how and why the school health services and school nursing developed. Discussion will include an exploration of the changing role of the school nurse to meet the new agenda and a consideration of the constraints on school nurses. The development of legal accountability for school nurses and an exploration of legal issues relating to the school-aged population will be considered. Finally, some of the challenges faced by school nurses since gaining the specialist community public health nursing (SCPHN) qualification will be explored.

Preventing childhood disease, the promotion and protection of child health, education and welfare are not new concepts although the development of statutory education and the school health service as a public health measure to promote and meet the health needs of school-aged children has come a long way since its inception 140 years ago. Health and education are inextricably linked and children cannot make the most of educational or employment opportunities if their health is impaired. Arguably, there is still a long way to go before all children and young people achieve their full health and educational potential but progress has been significant.

As with many other welfare developments in the UK, education and health care provision have their origins in the late nineteenth century. The following section uses a chronological approach to summarise significant statutory legislation relating to childhood education, the development of the school health service and school nursing including a consideration of the related drivers for change and implications.

History of the school health service

Up until the end of the nineteenth century education, health care and welfare for children was largely based on the ability of families to pay [1]. The attitude of British society towards the education of all children was mixed, whilst philanthropists argued for universal entitlement and some financed charitable schools; education was generally considered to be not only unnecessary but inappropriate for working class children as they were required for employment [2].

In 1870, in spite of fierce opposition the first legislation to establish a national and mainly free system of compulsory state education for all children in England and Wales was introduced and this required their entry into school from the age of five years to the age of eight years (Education Act 1870 (Forster's Education Act)). Similar provision was established in Northern Ireland and in Scotland (Scottish Education Act 1872). Political drivers for legislation were twofold: firstly, the need to educate people as citizens in the recently democratised and industrialised UK and secondly, in response to economic factors which required a literate and numerate workforce.

Interestingly, legislation in 1876 (Education Act 1876) placed a duty on parents to ensure that their children received elementary instruction in reading, writing and arithmetic although many families could not afford to send their children to school and it was not until 1890 (Elementary Education Act 1890) that grants became available to all schools to enable them to cease charging for basic elementary education. Many children did not attend school regularly and a report identified that sickness was the chief cause of absenteeism in schools and that illness was believed to be caused by neglect of care for the children's minor ailments and injuries [3].

From the end of the nineteenth century there was a gradual development of services to address the health and physical condition of children. The needs of children with special requirements were initially provided for in 1893 (Elementary Education (Blind and Deaf Children) Act 1893, Elementary Education (Defective and Epileptic Children) Act 1893), which empowered the newly formed local education authorities (LEAs) to set up special schools and classes for these children.

By 1899, there was a public outcry about the standard of child health and welfare. This was in response to a newspaper article which expressed concern about the appalling state of health of school-leavers enlisting for the army to fight in the Boer war (1899–1902).

> Reports in the national press claimed that two-thirds of the young men who volunteered to fight in the South African war had been rejected because of poor physique. [4, p. 45]

This provided a surprising catalyst for change and as a consequence of public concern, Parliament set up an Inter-departmental Committee [5] to report on the physical deterioration of the British nation. The report drew a shocking picture of the nation's children – high rates of infant and child mortality, infectious diseases and malnourished, thin, stunted children [6]. Similar findings were noted in France and Germany; however, they had already implemented health and nutritional programmes for school children. When the Lancet sent representatives to Paris, they found that free school meals of soup, meat and vegetables were being provided for each school child [4].

The Inter-departmental Committee report highlighted that good health in childhood was as fundamental to good health in adult life and proposed a series of public health reforms including the establishment of the school medical services [5]. In an effort to reduce the high infant and maternal mortality rates the report also recommended the registration of trained midwives and the provision of maternity care which was enacted in 1902 (Midwives Act 1902); however, similar legislation for the registration of nurses would not occur until 1919 (Nurses Registration Act 1919).

The twentieth century was a period of rapid development in both public health and personal health. The drivers for promoting child health were once again in direct response to a national need for healthy army recruits, 'as many as 60 per cent of boys were found to be unfit for duty because of poor eyesight, dental caries, heart disease and poor growth arising from poor childhood health' [7, p. 109].

Consequently, new legislation was implemented which focused on the health and development of the school child and enabled the provision of a nutritious meal for children whilst in school (The Education (Provision of Meals) Act 1906). Legislation in 1907 (Education (Administrative Provisions) Act 1907) identified the school as the most appropriate environment to focus on the health needs of the school-aged child and Section 13.1b of the Act established the school medical service which included the school entry medical inspection as a statutory right for all children; moreover, it allowed for additional inspections as necessary (Education (Administrative Provisions) Act 1907, Section 13.1b). The medical branch of the Board of Education was set up and its responsibilities included special educational treatment for handicapped children, establishing the school medical service, the provision of free school meals and at a later date the provision of free school milk and the organisation and inspection of physical training.

Maternity and infant welfare services were also developed at this time but were transferred to the Ministry of Health in 1919. The aim of these changes was primarily to reduce the infant and maternal mortality rates, to prevent any further deterioration in their health status and to promote the health and well-being of the child population to enable children to grow up and become healthy adults who could contribute to the society in which they lived. The public health focus of this service has always been based on health protection as well as health promotion although the service was generally prescriptive in its approach.

The role of unregistered and often untrained 'school nurses' at this time was predominantly in health and disease screening and working as assistants to the school medical officers [2] although there was the potential for opportunistic health promotion [8].

Under the Education Act 1918 (known as the Fisher Act) attending school became compulsory for all children up to the age of 14 years (Education Act 1918 (known as the Fisher Act)) and included the provision of additional ser- vices in schools such as medical inspections, nurseries and provision for pupils with special needs [2]. The Act allowed for the provision of medical treatment for primary-aged children, including ophthalmic and dental treatment, treat- ment for minor aliments, enlarged tonsils and adenoids. Increased central government involvement in education was a change in direction; however, the LEAs were given the power to direct the way in which the legislation was im- plemented (Legislation (www.opsi.gov.uk/legislation)). Industrialists reacted angrily to this legislation as it affected their productivity and economic well- being because they could no longer employ children under the age of 12 years, and children aged 12–14 years could only be employed for two hours a day. As a consequence of vociferous opposition and lobbying, a significant part of the legislation was not implemented (Education Act 1918).

Alongside changes in childhood education and health care provision there was increasing demand for improving the provision of medical, nursing and midwifery services by establishing a national minimal standard of education, preparation and training. Health visiting originated in 1852 through the de- velopment of the Manchester and Salford Reform Association and Florence Nightingale was instrumental in setting up national health visitor training in the 1890s [9]. The quality of midwifery care was also variable throughout the UK; therefore, legislation to standardise midwifery education, training and practice was established and made midwifery a national registered qualifi- cation. The Central Midwives Board was established as the regulatory body responsible for the education, training, conduct and performance of midwives (Midwives Act 1902).

Legislation in 1919 included the establishment of the General Nursing Coun- cil as the regulatory body responsible for the education, training, conduct and performance of nurses (The Nurses' Registration Act 1919). This was a significant development in the UK as the majority of 'nurses' including school nurses were untrained women who developed their skills whilst working in the role. It is argued that Florence Nightingale was one of the principal movers for this legislation as well as political acknowledgement of the crucial role that nurses played during the World War I (1914-1918) [10].

Activity 5.1

Consider the following:
What were the driving forces for the introduction of the school medical service and what was the role of the school nurse at this time?
What preparation did the school nurse have for undertaking this role?

In the 1920s, with the development of the welfare state the subjects of health and education became sensitive, social, political and economic issues. The government created a series of commissions of enquiry to explore the issues and propose ways of improving these services. In 1944, legislation replaced previous education laws and for the first time adopted a child-centred approach and acknowledged the interrelationship between the child, its family and the wider community.

> It shall be the duty of the local education authority for every area, so far as their powers extend, to continue towards the spiritual, mental and physical development of the community. [Education Act 1944 Part II, 7 (Education Act 1944. Commonly known as the Butler Act).]

Section 48 of the Education Act 1944 required all education authorities not only to provide regular medical inspections for all children but also to make arrangements for medical treatment (Education Act 1944 (commonly known as the Butler Act), Section 48). This was a significant development because of the social upheaval of the time due to the World War II (1939-1945) where children evacuated from deprived industrialised areas were found to be infested, generally unwell and some had severe behavioural problems as a consequence of political neglect and educational deprivation [2].

The School Health Service (Handicapped Pupils) Regulations 1945 outlined the responsibilities of the health visitor within the school health services in line with the Education Act 1944 (The School Health Service (Handicapped Pupils) Regulations 1945). Health visitors were registered nurses with additional midwifery or obstetric qualifications and had completed a post-registration nursing course in public health nursing – health visiting [10].

Health visitor autonomy in developing health promotion with the school-aged population was acknowledged in law even though the majority of their work focused on families with pre-school-aged children. This was in stark contrast to the role of the school nurse which was specifically with the school-aged population but this role was arguably less autonomous and variable in its nature. School nurses were employed mainly by the LEAs and their work focused mainly on disease screening and they worked under the direction of either the medical officers or the schools.

The National Health Service and post-World War II

Following the World War II, the National Health Service (NHS) Act 1946 was implemented in 1948 which was a major development in the universal provision of health care (National Health Service Act 1946). Section 24 of the Act emphasised the public health nature of the work of the health visitor regarding health promotion, disease preventive and social aspects of the role including working with schools and the school-aged population (National Health Service Act 1946, Section 24); however, the role of the school nurse had not been acknowledged.

As a result of government concern about the high infant mortality rates and the incidence of childhood illnesses and diseases in 1956 the Jameson report reviewed the role of the health visitor and made significant proposals for the improvement of the syllabus and educational preparation for health visitors [11]. The Jameson report promoted the concept of health visitors providing a public service which spanned across the lifespan and one of its recommendations was for health visitors to play a larger part in health education in schools [9].

As a consequence of the 1945 and 1946 Acts and the Jameson report health visitors were designated as the named school nurses for nurseries, primary and secondary schools in England and Wales [11] even though a significant amount of the screening work in schools was undertaken by NHS-employed clinic nurses who fed back their findings to the health visitors. Furthermore, LEA employed school nurses who were based in the schools and had developed positive relationships with both the school children and teachers could not undertake health education sessions as this was deemed to be the responsibility of the health visitor. This situation was very frustrating for all concerned and continued in many areas of the UK until the 1990s.

Thirty years of research analysing the role of the health visitor found that the majority of the work concentrated on children from birth to five years old, so arguably there was little opportunity to develop their public health role with the school-aged population. There are numerous reasons for this restriction including NHS priorities, funding arrangements for the provision of services, the health visitor's job description, carrying a large caseload, working in areas of deprivation and having a high prevalence of vulnerable children on their caseloads. The implications of this for the school-aged population were significant and the recommendations of both the Jameson report and the Council for the Education and Training of Health Visitor (CETHV) 1965 syllabus were rarely realised in practice, so the public health and health promotion needs of the school-aged population were largely ignored.

Changes in schools

In 1965, the Labour government issued a circular which encouraged LEAs in England and Wales to move away from the selective form of secondary schooling and adopt a more comprehensive approach [12]. The government-appointed committee in 1967 recommended the end of selective grouping of children by their abilities ('streaming') and a return to a more child-centred and humanitarian approaches to primary schooling which was evident prior to 1939 [13].

By 1988, legislation required every school to provide a nine-subject national curriculum and to ensure that every child attending school had the full range of the national curriculum (Education Reform Act 1988). This provided an exciting opportunity for school nurses to work closely with teachers to develop child health promotion within this framework.

The responsibility for the school health service, the employment of medical officers and school nurses came within the remit of LEAs; however, this was found to be both isolating and problematic, as other health colleagues were employed by the NHS resulting in liaison, referrals and meeting difficulties. In 1974, school nurses and medical officers transferred their employment to the NHS although LEAs became responsible for the coordination of all child health services, but by 1982, this responsibility was also transferred to the district health authorities as a result of the 'Patient First' reorganisation (National Health Service (Reorganisation) Act 1974).

> the aim of this new health service for children was to bring together health professionals ... in order to provide preschool, school health, hospital and specialist services. [8, p. 110]

Some LEAs chose to employ school nurses directly and this situation persists in areas of the UK although their role remains significantly different to that of school nurses employed by the NHS [14]. The separation of education and health has created some relationship difficulties as the school health service is no longer directly under the control of the LEA. Trying to gain access to the schools, school children and appropriate facilities for school medicals, screening tests and health promotion activities has on occasion been a challenge for some school nurses. This requires effective multi-agency working and interpersonal relationships with the school staff to maximise the effectiveness and efficiency of both services. Whilst the majority of schools value the contribution of the school health service and school nurses there are clearly educational priorities that take precedence.

In 1976, the court report acknowledged the difficulties inherent in agencies working together and cooperating to meet the needs of the child and stressed that the connection between health and education was vital for child health [15].

The report argued that child health should be at the centre of planning and rather than having all services in the school they should also be available in the community and in the children's own homes; however, this approach was not implemented and in 1995, the Polnay report again reiterated this crucial point when identifying the health needs of the school-aged children and making very detailed recommendations for the provision of school health services [16].

Legislative aspects

When considering the development of school nursing the effects of legislation and policies had a significant impact on the direction of the service. This is particularly relevant when the regulatory body changed and established the potential for specialist practice in school nursing through the Nurses, Midwives and Health Visitors Act 1979.

> The act has generated a larger professional base, and has made progress in equating the governance of nurses, midwives and health visitors with that of doctors in key respects of autonomy, registration, specified training and standards of practice. [17, p. 161]

Following deliberation, lobbying from nurses and protests regarding the development of community nursing in 1994 the UKCC published their standards for qualified and registered nurses, midwives and health visitors known as the post-registration education and practice project (PREPP). This included a wide range of requirements for professional development and competence for all registered practitioners and specifically included the reform of community nursing education [18] (see Chapter 9).

This had significant implications for the development of school nursing as it enabled universities and approved higher education institutions to set up post-registration nursing degree courses in community nursing which included a UKCC-recorded specialist community practitioner qualification for eight discrete areas of community nursing including school nursing. This created a route for school nurses to achieve academic and clinical qualifications in specialist professional practice and was an important milestone. At last there was acknowledgement from the UKCC that school nursing was an important area of community nursing warranting specialist knowledge, skills and expertise.

School nurses whether they were employed by LEAs, health authorities, independent schools or charitable organisations were required to be registered with the UKCC as nurses [19]. However, the level of nurse registration or what branch of nursing the school nurse was registered under was not specified by either the employers or the UKCC. There is no available data identifying what post-registration qualifications, if any, these school nurses had. Arguably, many school nurses working in a range of settings had no specific education, training or preparation in child health, health promotion or public health nursing to undertake this unique role. This was in stark contrast to health visiting where only UKCC-registered health visitors could be employed in that specific role following an approved post-registration course [18].

Very few employers required school nurses to have specific qualifications so the availability of specialist practitioner courses in school nursing received a mixed reception amongst employers. Before agreeing to releasing school nurses on to these courses employers would have to consider the cost and implications for their service provision.

The National Assembly for Wales (NAW) saw the value in developing the knowledge, skills and expertise of their health care workforce and agreed to fund the community nursing degree courses for health visitors, district nurses, practice nurses, community learning disability nurses, community children's nurses, community mental health nurses and school nurses (National Assembly for Wales (now called Welsh Assembly Government; www.assemblywales.org)). The NAW also agreed to reimburse NHS trusts who released these nurses to undertake the course to enable them to employ replacement staff for the duration of the course [20] – this is commonly known as backfill replacement costs. The availability of funding for England, Scotland and Northern Ireland was variable, with students in some areas having to self-fund the course.

England, Scotland and Northern Ireland provided a range of courses for school nurses but in Wales there were no degree courses specifically focusing on the professional practice of school nursing until the commencement of the BSc (Hons) in community health nursing at the University of Glamorgan in 1999. This included a school nursing pathway and enabled successful graduates to record their SPQ with the UKCC. Whilst the course was made available to all school nurses, eligibility for NAW funding was restricted to those employed by the NHS and disappointingly to date, there have not been any non-NHS-employed school nurses accessing the course. Within two years, school nursing degree courses were established throughout Wales.

The Cumberlege report

At this time, a number of policies came into effect which had an impact on child health and service provision. The Cumberlege report [21] reviewed the way in which community nursing was organised and envisaged teams of nurses with a mixture of skills and expertise working together to meet the health needs of the population. The need for partnership between all professional impacting on the health of a given population was emphasised and focused on moving these teams away from general practice (GP). Thirteen recommendations were made and included three arguments for moving nursing teams away from GP.

(1) District nurses, health visitors and school nurses working in a team could be a major force for change and improvement in community health services.
(2) Apart from other benefits, the neighbourhood nursing service would bring school nursing in from the periphery of primary care arguing that the needs of a neighbourhood's children would be brought into focus and would make it easier to take a more integrated, family-based approach to the health care of children and young people.

(3) Following an assessment of particular health needs the neighbourhood nursing team could bring the issues to the GP who would be able to access more nursing skills than would be traditionally available.

GP reluctance to accept these changes and lose control of the nursing teams resulted in the report not being fully implemented, although it could be argued that when developing the family nursing model in Scotland the recommendations of Cumberlege were considered [22].

> ### Activity 5.2
>
> - Consider what were the driving forces for the professional development of the school nurse?
> - What preparation did the school nurse have to undertake this role?

School nursing in the twenty-first century

Since 1974 the National Health Service Act has been the subject to a constant stream of political reform. Recently, the numerous NHS Acts have been consolidated into the NHS Act 2006 which came into effect in March 2007, but effects little change. [23, p. 20]

As a result of devolution in Wales, Scotland and Northern Ireland, child health services have changed throughout the UK and the school health services have developed slightly differently in each country. In many areas of the UK the stereotypical image of a school nurse based in a single school working with a wide job description has been replaced by a school nurse employed by the NHS who has responsibilities for a number of schools and has a more focused public health and health promotion role. However, the Royal College of Nursing (RCN) survey identified five main categories of school nurse defined by their job title and location of work and the variations in the role [14]. Whilst being mindful of addressing local needs this survey highlighted that a more universal standard of school nursing was required [14].

The chief nursing officer in 2006 [24] acknowledged that school nurses are well placed to deliver on a range of public health outcomes and have two key responsibilities:

- To assess, protect and promote the health and well-being of school-aged children and young people
- To offer advice, care and treatment to individuals and groups of children, young people and the adults who care for them [25]

This was a watershed in the development of school nursing as it publicised to head - teachers, governors and others that school nurses are a valuable resource and the actual and potential areas of child public health that school nursing should be engaging in.

Throughout the UK the role of the school nurse has changed significantly over the past 140 years to one where she or he works as an autonomous public health practitioner. As the scope of practice increases so does the demand for professional and legal accountability by measuring the effectiveness and efficiency of the service provided as well as the competency of the school nurse. This is why the incorporation of clinical governance, reflection, clinical supervision and accountability for practice are crucial in the development of school nursing.

Accountability

Accountability and school nurses

The Nursing and Midwifery Council (NMC) states in the code that:

> As a professional, you are personally accountable for actions and omissions in your practice and must always be able to justify your decisions. [26, p. 1]

Activity 5.3

- Consider the purpose of holding school nurses accountable for their actions and write down what you believe you are accountable for.
- Does the level or breadth of accountability differ according to your grade?

Accountability is therefore defined as being answerable for your personal acts and omissions to a higher authority with whom you have a legal relationship. [27, p. 32]

School nurses are personally accountable for their behaviour and this includes ethical, moral and legal dimensions. The moral dimension is one of the reasons why reflective practice is so important for school nurses. Chapter 2 identified that all SCPHNs are legally and professionally accountable for their actions and omissions so the discussion below will focus specifically on accountability for school nurses.

Griffith and Tengnah [27] explain that accountability has four functions:

- **A protective function**: To protect the public if someone falls below the standard required of them in law.
- **A deterrent function**: To act as a deterrent by discouraging nurses to act illegally or unprofessionally.

- **A regulatory function**: To regulate behaviour by making it clear the standard of conduct and competence that registered nurses must comply with.
- **An educative function**: To educate society and practitioners about what the standards of professional practice are.

Ignorantia legis neminem excusat (*Ignorance of the law excuses no one*)

It is not acceptable for a school nurse to plead ignorance as she may not escape liability for breaking the law just because she was unaware of it. People have a presumed knowledge of the law so a school nurse must know the laws that relate to her practice. Knowledge of related law is a positive thing and can prevent harm so that your actions protect society, children, young people and their families, colleagues, the profession and yourself. Dimond [28] states that the four arenas of legal accountability are:

- To the public through criminal law and the criminal courts
- To the patient through civil law and the civil courts
- To the employer through the contract of employment and the employment tribunal
- To the profession through the NMC [26] code and in disciplinary proceedings before the committees of the NMC

School nurses are legally accountable to the public, to the school child or young person and their families, to the profession, their employer and the schools; however, it is unusual for a school nurse to be called to account in all four arenas at the same time although the potential is there. Whilst anyone may have to justify their actions to others the standards used in law to measure a person's actions varies considerably between these four arenas of law.

Accountability to the public

School nurses are subject to the same statutory laws (Acts of Parliament) as other members of society, for example, all householders must ensure that their premises are safe for visitors and if a law is broken then action in the criminal courts may be the consequence (Occupiers Liability Act 1957 and Occupiers Liability Act 1984) [29]. School Nurses are also subject to specific laws relating to their professional practice, for example, during childhood vaccination sessions a range of legislation apply (Health and Safety at Work etc. Act 1974, Medicines Act 1968, Children Act 1989 and Children Act 2004).

Criminal charges in relation to school nursing specifically are thankfully rare; however, charges against other nurses working with children are not unheard of, for example Beverley Allitt, an Enrolled Nurse working on a children's ward was brought before the High Court and found guilty of murdering four children, attempting to murder three other children and of causing grievous bodily harm to six other children. She was given nine life sentences and minimum of

30 years imprisonment [30]. The consequences of her actions meant that she was also brought to account in civil law, employment law and professional law.

Accountability to the school child or young person

Children are the focus of the public health role of the school nurse and are a particularly vulnerable group in society. Statutory law acknowledges this and sets out clear standards and responsibilities for all agencies involved in caring for children and in safeguarding and protecting them from harm. The principles contained in the United Nations Convention on the Rights of the Child is the first legally binding international instrument to incorporate the full range of human rights for children and young people in UK law [31].

The core principles of the Convention are:

- Non-discrimination
- Devotion to the best interests of the child
- The right to life
- Survival and development
- Respect for the views of the child

The Convention protects children's rights by setting standards in health care, education, and legal, civil and social services and most of the articles were incorporated into UK law. For example, Article 19 of the Convention states that children have the right to protection from abuse and the Children Act 1989 and Children Act 2004 provide the legislative framework for this. As a consequence everyone working with children has a legal obligation to promote and uphold children's rights; this includes school nurses who have a key role in safeguarding children and promoting their health, welfare and autonomy.

Autonomy, consent and the child

Respect for autonomy is valued as an ethical principle in nursing, midwifery and SCPHN practice and practitioners should have a working knowledge of legal and ethical issues relating to autonomy and consent to treatment [26, 32]. See summary of the definition and requirements of consent in Box 5.1.

Box 5.1 Consent

Consent can be defined as 'a patient's agreement for a health profes-sional to provide care' [33].
For consent to be valid the patient must:

- Be competent to take a particular decision
- Have received sufficient information to take it
- Not be acting under duress

School nurses undertake a range of public health, health promotion and health care interventions with children and young people therefore it is essential that any advice, treatment or care is undertaken within the confines of the law. Obtaining consent and upholding confidentiality are an essential requirement and mentally competent adults are able to make autonomous decisions regarding their health and welfare [33]. The development of autonomy is a gradual process and children and young people require support and protection in law until they are sufficiently mature enough to make informed choices. The principles governing the legal capacities of children, the responsibilities of parents and the limits of state intervention have largely been developed in the context of medical decision-making as health is the most basic and essential consideration in protecting child welfare [23]. Courts recognise that children are not autonomous adults but do have rights to give their own consent to treatment as they develop and mature [34]. School nurses must be aware of the law and their responsibilities to children regarding consent and confidentiality.

Consent and the 16 and 17 year old

The Family Law Reform Act 1969 defines an adult as a person aged 18 years or over, so a minor is a person who has not yet achieved her or his 18th birthday (Family Law Reform Act 1969, Section 1).

This Act also acknowledges that 16 and 17 year olds have sufficient autonomy to give their own consent to medical, surgical and dental treatment (Family Law Reform Act 1969, Section 1, Section 8(1)) and investigations (Family Law Reform Act 1969, Section 1, Section 8(2)) without reference to their parents. This presumption is also included in the Mental Health Act 1983. The Family Law Reform Act 1969 does not prevent an unconscious 16 or 17 year old from being given life-saving treatment in an emergency [28] or the parents of an incapacitated young person from giving consent by proxy (Family Law Reform Act 1969, Section 8(3)).

One area of concern is when a 16 or 17 year old refuses to give consent for treatment or care. Challenges to their autonomy have resulted in legal action, for example, in Re W (a minor: medical treatment) [1992] the Court of Appeal overruled W's refusal to receive life-saving treatment [35]. Equally, since the implementation of the Mental Health Act 2007 in October 2008, parents can no longer give consent for their 16–17 year old to be admitted to a psychiatric unit for treatment (Mental Health Act 2007). So whilst adults are able to determine whether or not to receive treatment the same standards do not apply to 16–17 year olds who are deemed to be autonomous if they agree to have treatment but not if they refuse.

Consent and the child under 16 years old

Where a child lacks capacity to consent, then any one person with 'parental responsibility' or by the court can give that consent on behalf of the child (by proxy). Parental responsibility is a legal concept introduced by the Children Act 1989 and is defined as,

All the rights, duties, powers, responsibility and authority which by law a parent of a child has in relation to the child and his property.

(Children Act 1989, Section 3(1))

Activity 5.4

Consider who has parental responsibility and what it means?
What are the limitations of parental responsibility?

Automatic parental responsibility is conferred upon the mother of the child (Children Act 1989, Section 3(1), Section 2) and on the father if he was married to the mother at the time of the child's birth or shortly after (Children Act 1989, Section 3(1), Section 1). Single fathers did not have parental responsibility as an automatic right and arguably most of these fathers did not realise it. From a school nurse's perspective this was problematic when trying to gain consent for immunisation or any other health care intervention. This situation remained for 12 years until the Adoption and Children Act 2002 was implemented in December 2003 (England and Wales) so that the unmarried father if he jointly registers the birth with the mother also has parental responsibility (Adoption and Children Act 2002). School nurses need to be aware that this change in parental responsibility is not retrospective so does not apply to unmarried fathers of children born before December 2003.

Other people may also have parental responsibility such as legal guardians, person(s) with a residence order, adoptive parents (when the birth mother permanently loses parental responsibility as part of the adoption process). Parental responsibility is not lost when parents divorce and most parents retain this when a child is accommodated by the local authority or police.

The welfare principle means that parental responsibility is only valid if the parent is acting in the best interests of the child.

Parental responsibility diminishes as children mature and ceases when a child reaches 18 years of age in England, Wales and Northern Ireland. In Scotland parental responsibility ceases when a child reaches 16 but parents can still give guidance until they are 18 [36]. Children grow and develop at varying rates and as the precedent from *Gillick* v *West Norfolk and Wisbech Area Health Authority* [1986] identified competent minors can consent to treatment or care on their own behalf if the child could achieve sufficient comprehension to understand completely the treatment proposed, with both its benefits and side effects [37]. However, they still cannot refuse treatment which may be needed in life-saving situations. Getting the child to agree to the involvement of the parents in the decision-making process is desirable but not always achievable.

Lord Fraser (Law Lord) developed a set of criteria that must apply when health professionals are offering contraceptive services to minors less than 16 years of age. The criteria are used to establish the competence of the minor. An important consideration for school nurses when assessing competence using the Fraser guidelines is that it is not an on/off procedure, a child may be deemed competent for a specific form of treatment but not for another, and therefore the assessment would need carried out on each occasion. See Box 5.2 for a summary of the Fraser guidelines.

Box 5.2   The Fraser guidelines

(1) The young person understands the health professional's advice
(2) The health professional cannot persuade the young person to inform his or her parents or allow the doctor to inform the parents that he or she is seeking contraceptive advice
(3) The young person is very likely to begin or continue having intercourse with or without contraceptive treatment
(4) Unless he or she receives contraceptive advice or treatment, the young person's physical or mental health (or both) is likely to suffer
(5) The young person's best interests require the health professional to give contraceptive advice, treatment or both without parental consent

Department of Health [38]. Reproduced with permission.

School nurses need to be aware that a child who is deemed to be a mature minor is also entitled to an obligation of confidentiality, unless the school nurse believes that maintaining confidentiality may be harmful for that child or others.

Safeguarding children

Because of the nature of their role school nurses may be the first to identify that a child is distressed or at risk of being harmed. The school nurse must have the knowledge, skills and expertise to deal with the situation effectively and, if appropriate, implement the child protection procedures. A school nurse who does not honour the requirements set out in the Children Act 1989, the Children Act 2004 or the Local Child Protection procedures would be liable.

Safeguarding children and young people is a major part of the school nurse's role. In line with the Chief Nursing Officer's review in 2004 [39] there are now a wider range of nurses taking up posts as child protection nurses, a number of whom have a school nurse background. School nurses can act as key workers in ensuring the needs of the child is foremost and the model of 'team around the child' is one that is increasing.

Children and young people in the looked after system are considered already vulnerable, disadvantaged and probably living in poverty and could possibly be viewed as a group, which, due to their circumstances, are unable to respond to health promotion messages. Mayall in 1976 (cited in Ref. [40]) describes a model in which at one end of a very long continuum is the school of thought that ill health is viewed as being a direct consequence of poverty and at the other end, the view that in whatever social circumstances individuals may find themselves in, they have the ability to change their health behaviour. Of course, linked intrinsically with this is the individual development and maturity of the child or young person, and their ability to make healthy choices within the family unit in which they live.

Vulnerable groups

Children and young people are one of the most vulnerable groups within the community, and they have public health needs that are significantly different to those of adults [39]. However, some children and young people are deemed to be more vulnerable than others. It is estimated that approximately three million children in England alone are vulnerable. See Box 5.3 for categories of vulnerability.

Box 5.3 Vulnerable children

Those being looked after by local authorities
Young offenders
Children of refugees or asylum seekers
Those living in poverty
Those who misuse substances
Those who have behavioural difficulties
Homeless young people
Those with disabilities
Young teenage parents
Travelling families
Those from ethnic minority backgrounds
Young carers
Young men in general also require additional input from health and
    youth services

From a school nursing perspective active recruitment of male school nurses and those from different ethnic and cultural backgrounds may help to engage some of these children and young people. Appleton [41] suggests that vulnerable school-aged children and young people are increasingly defined as those where there is concern about their welfare. But whatever the definition vulnerable children and young people are more at risk of suffering negative outcomes in relation to their health in its broadest sense, i.e. mentally, physically and socially.

DeBell and Everett [42] highlight that school nurses are clearly able to recognise distress in children, and this can be particularly highlighted in relation to child protection and mental health issues. These are two key areas, which are both complex and demanding areas of practice. The school nurse may be the first person the child or young person has either disclosed allegations of abuse to or has sought a 'listening ear' to share their physical and emotional distress. In these situations the school nurse can play a significant role both in supporting and safeguarding the child as well as acting as their advocate.

Young people not attending mainstream school

There are children and young people who do not regularly attend mainstream school who may have been excluded or who are educated at home for a variety of reasons. They may be disadvantaged further in that they are not offered an equitable service in comparison to their peer group in the same area. Those not attending school are considered to be more at risk of becoming involved in risk-taking behaviours, which are detrimental to health [43] and are often more vulnerable who still need access to high quality, accurate information. Children and young people who are looked after by local authorities are ten times more likely to be excluded from school [44], which has a significant impact on their health, employment opportunities and economic well-being.

'Hard-to-reach' groups

The use of technology such as websites and text messaging are vital methods of communicating with today's young people particularly those deemed to be 'hard to reach'. However, this term in itself is debatable as it is professionals who believe such groups are considered 'hard to reach'. But should this be turned on its head and may be it is the professionals and services who are actually 'hard to access' by some client groups such as young people not attending school? Therefore, we need to take positive steps to develop and provide services that meet people where they are in a way that is more suitable to them. It is important to start from the perspective of the vulnerable children/groups themselves, in designing appropriate services that meet their specific health needs. It is the quality of the intervention and its appropriateness and acceptability to the client group that are crucial.

Activity 5.5

Consider how you see your role/your team's role in supporting children and young people outside of the school setting. Justify your involvement and consider how you could provide evidence to commissioners of your/ your team's effectiveness.

Working together

Article 24 of the United Nations Convention on the Rights of the Child states that children have a right to the highest obtainable standard of health possible and this requires adequate health care to meet their needs. Article 24.2(e) [45] includes the duty to ensure that parents and children have information regarding child health and nutrition. This requires school nurses to work closely with teachers, school governors and other agencies to formulate and implement understandable, developmentally appropriate health promotion programmes which enable and empower children, young people and their parents to improve their nutritional status.

Civil law focuses on the rights of an individual to redress. If an individual believes he or she has been harmed then he or she (or his or her representative) is entitled to make a claim and take legal action against the person who he or she believes caused that harm. The laws of tort include issues such as consent, confidentiality, trespass and negligence and if the person proves the case then he or she will be given financial compensation from the person who caused the harm. In order to succeed in a case of negligence there are four elements that need to be established:

- The defendant has a duty of care to the claimant
- There is a breach in the standard of the duty of care owed
- This breach has caused reasonably foreseeable harm
- The harm of which the victim complains was caused by that breach [28, p. 9]

All four of the above elements have to be established for a person to win his or her case and be compensated. The number of negligence cases brought before the courts has escalated and the time spent and the cost of going to court can be significant for either party if they lose the case. The cost of having to pay compensation in a negligence case creates a drain on the NHS budget and a resulting loss of public trust in the competence of NHS staff to provide high standards of care.

In the NHS clinical negligence claims have a potential value of some 4 billion pounds. In 2006-7 alone some £579.3 million was paid out in connection with clinical negligence claims [46].

A school nurse has a duty of care not only to school-aged children and young people in their care but also to anyone else affected by their actions or omissions, including colleagues, school staff and parents. However, it would be unreasonable for a school nurse who is part of a team covering a cluster of primary schools and a comprehensive to be individually accountable to all of these children at all times. *Donoghue* v *Stevenson* [1932] [47] established that we all have a duty of care to anyone affected by our reasonably foreseeable actions. For example, if a school nurse gives unsafe advice on the management of anaphylaxis which results in a child being harmed then the school nurse may be liable and could be sued by the child or his or her parent.

It is difficult to measure the standard of care given by school nurses because the role varies enormously depending on the employer and job description; however, the precedent set by *Bolam* v *Friern* [1957] [48] establishes the reasonable standard expected by someone exercising and performing that particular art, so a school nurse would be compared with that which is reasonably expected of another school nurse. The Bolam test does not expect the highest standard of practice just the reasonable standard, although school nurses should be striving for excellence, and it could be argued that the Bolam standard is not set high enough as highlighted in *Bolitho* v *City and Hackney Health Authority* [1998] [49].

The precedence in *Wilsher* v *Essex Health Authority* [1988] [50] acknowledges that inexperience is no defence, for example a school nurse carrying out vaccinations is required to be safe whether or not she has additional qualifications or has been qualified for five days or five years. If a person accepts a role it is his or her responsibility to ensure that he or she can carry it out safely. Equally, it is also reasonable to expect that any additional education and training should be reflected in the standard of that school nurse's practice and subsequently the expectations of employers, schools, school-aged children and the public would be greater. The accountability of the school nurse to the child would include all the activities required to protect that child from harm and to promote that child's health and well-being. Acquiring the appropriate knowledge, skills and understanding of all these issues are essential to protect the child and also protects the school nurse from litigation.

Accountability to the employer

Employment law originates from statutory law and the school nurse is accountable to her employer through the contract of employment whether employed by the NHS, LEA, Independent school or charitable organisation.

An employer also has a duty of care to his or her employee; therefore, an NHS trust would be vicariously liable for a school nurse's work because the trust appointed her and is responsible for ensuring that she has the expected level of knowledge, skills and expertise and that a safe standard of work is provided. The employer is also responsible for ensuring that all staff has an opportunity to attend study days or practice sessions where new pieces of equipment are introduced.

Consideration also needs to be given to the contract of employment, terms and conditions of service and any job description as the NHS trust may not be vicarious liable (indirect liability) if a school nurse works outside her job description. Accountability to the employer is the arena where most nurses are called to justify their actions for two reasons: firstly, children, parents and colleagues are more likely to complain to the employer rather than take legal action; secondly, the burden of proof in employment law is lower than that required in the civil and the criminal courts.

Employment law only requires that an employer hold an honest and genuine belief that an employee is guilty of misconduct based on the outcome of a reasonable investigation [51].

Accountability to the profession

The NMC was set up by Parliament to regulate the profession, set standards, approve courses and hold practitioners accountable for their actions as a way of firstly ensuring that the public and patients are not harmed and secondly providing redress to people who have been harmed (Nurses, Midwives and Health Visitors Act 1997; Nursing and Midwifery Order 2001).

In order to practice the school nurse needs to be registered with the NMC, and affirm accountability to the profession and agree to abide by the NMC code of professional conduct which is the recognised ethical code determining the standard of practice [26]. Registrants must affirm that they are keeping up to date with their practice and meet the NMC PREP requirements [52] if a school nurse is found by the NMC Conduct and Competence Committee to be guilty of breaking the clauses within the code then her name can be removed from the register.

A professional law case that subsequently became a civil law case involved a school nurse administering childhood vaccinations in a school, *Hefferon* v *Committee of the UKCC* [1988] [53]. During a vaccination session, the school nurse erroneously injected a child who was not due for vaccination and she immediately reported the error to the medical officer and her line manager. The child was examined by the doctor and was apparently unharmed. The school nurse's line manager reported the incident to the UKCC and she was referred to the Professional Conduct Committee. Allegations of professional misconduct were made and evidence presented by the school nurse's manager and others were compared with the UKCC Code of professional conduct [19]. Hefferon was found guilty of professional misconduct on a number of counts and the decision was made to remove her name from the UKCC register so that she could no longer practice as a nurse.

Hefferon subsequently took her case to the civil courts. The High Court established that the laws of natural justice had not been applied during the Professional Conduct Committee and Hefferon had not been given the opportunity to state her case, present any evidence to support her actions or challenge the evidence presented against her [53]. The decision of the UKCC to remove her name from the register was subsequently quashed.

As a consequence of the Hefferon case and other concerns about the statutory functions of the UKCC an independent review was ordered by the government and undertaken by JM Consulting who in their 1999 report made recommendations for changing the statutory role, functions and accountability of the regulatory body for nurses, midwives and health visitors [54]. The government accepted the findings and produced a consultation paper [55]. This led to new legislation causing in the dissolution of the UKCC being replaced by the Nursing and Midwifery Council in April 2002 (Health Act 1999, Section 60). This is discussed more fully in Chapter 2; however, the specific implications of incorporating school nursing as a registerable qualification within the SCPHN will now be considered [56].

The development of the role of the SCPHN – school nurse

There remains a significant variation in the provision of health care for the school-aged population and the role of the school nurse employed by the LEA, the NHS, Independent Schools and charitable organisations vary significantly.

The RCN undertook a census survey of school nurses in 2005 and identified that the roles of school nurses varied significantly according to their job title and where they worked [14]. School nurses employed by education did not provide the same type or level of service as those employed by the NHS. The role of the school nurse employed by the LEA frequently included non-nursing duties such as collecting dinner money, photocopying, health and safety officer and first-aid responsibilities whilst those employed by the NHS were specifically involved in child health surveillance and health promotion work.

When the NMC Standards of proficiency for SCPHN were introduced school nurses were arguably ecstatic that they finally had the opportunity to gain national recognition for their role and the regulatory body for the profession was condoning a graduate programme of education leading to a registerable qualification for school nurses as specialists in public health school nursing [56].

The implementation of the course was not without problem as the standards set for the different fields of SCPHN practice were the same even though the defined areas of practice were different [57]. For decades the health visiting courses had required health visitor/community practice teachers (PTs) to support and assess students throughout their clinical placements. These PTs had specific qualifications to undertake their roles and their NHS employers supported them in clinical practice in two ways: firstly, by agreeing to give them a reduced case load and secondly, by rewarding them financially and setting them at a higher grade than their generic health visiting colleagues so that they could concentrate their efforts of facilitating learning in the clinical environment.

In sharp contrast previous school nursing courses had facilitators to support them in practice. These experienced school nurses did not have any specific qualifications to take on the teaching and learning support role and did not receive any financial reward for their involvement in the learning process. Section 7 of the NMC standards established the PT requirements for all fields and stated that by 2007 all PTs had to meet the standards required in the 2004 document [58]. This was problematic for the school nursing pathway of the SCPHN course as nationally there were very few SCPHN school nurses who met the criteria required to become PTs. As a result many universities requested a process of deferment in meeting the criteria until sufficient numbers of SCPHN school nurses could undertake the PT training before supporting students. The NMC acknowledged that there was inequity and establishes the opportunities to apply for deferment until 2010 [59].

The second area of inequity between PTs in health visiting and school nursing occurred within NHS trusts as SCPHN - school nurse PTs were not initially given a higher grade or reduced workload to enable them to fulfil their PT requirements. This is now being addressed although progress is slow and there remains a significant discrepancy between the NHS agenda for change grade that NHS trusts implement for SCPHN - school nurse PTs and SCPHN - health visitor PTs [60].

Summary

This chapter has reviewed the historical development of the school health service and explored how the public health role of the school nurse has evolved. The relevant drivers for change, legislation and social policy were considered to explore how the service evolved to meet the new public health agenda. The accountability of the school nurse to the child, society, the profession and the employer was discussed and the development of the public health function of school nurses explored. Consideration of the educational preparation, training and support required to enable school nurses to develop their role was included and identified the historical inequity in the educational preparation of school nurses.

The NMC as regulator for the profession has acknowledged that school nursing is a registerable qualification and while disparity in child health, education and life chances continues there is a need for the school health services, school nursing and public health approaches to meet the health needs of the younger generation. The future for school nursing is robustly optimistic, particularly now that government has recognised the untapped potential and opportunities for promoting and protecting the health of school-aged children and young people. The next chapter will consider the current situation relating to school nursing practice and how the public health agenda is developing.

References

1 Baly M. The setting. In: Nash W, Thruston M, eds. *Health at School: Caring for the Whole Child.* Oxford: Butterworth, 1985, pp. 2-16.

2 Webber I. Professions and school nursing. In: Symonds A, Kelly A, eds. *The Social Construction of Community Care.* Basingstoke: Macmillan, 1998.

3 Zaiger D. Historical perspectives of school nursing. In: Selekman J, ed. *School Nursing: A Comprehensive Text.* Philadelphia: F. A. Davis Company, 2006, pp. 3-24.

4 Barker DJP. Obesity and early life. *Obesity Reviews* 2007; **8**(Suppl 1): 45-9.

5 Inter-departmental Committee on Physical Deterioration. *Report of the Inter-departmental Committee on Physical Deterioration.* London: HMSO, 1904.

6 Lightfoot J, Bines W. Working to keep school children healthy: the complementary roles of school staff and school nurses. *Journal of Public Health Medicine* 2000; **22**(1): 74–80.

7 Leff S, Leff V. The school as location for health promotion. In: DeBell D, ed. *Public Health Practice and the School-Age Population.* London: Hodder Arnold, 2007, pp. 93–130.

8 DeBell D, ed. *Public Health Practice and The School-Age Population.* London: Hodder Arnold, 2007.

9 Porter E. Public health and health visiting. In: Robotham A, Frost M, eds. *Health Visiting: Specialist Community Public Health Nursing.* Edinburgh: Elsevier Churchill Livingstone, 2005.

10 Robotham A. The profession of health visiting in the 21st century. In: Robotham A, Frost M, eds. *Health Visiting: Specialist Community Public Health Nursing.* Edinburgh: Elsevier Churchill Livingstone, 2005, pp. 5–27.

11 Ministry of Health. *An Inquiry into Health Visiting.* London: HMSO, 1956.

12 Department of Education and Science. *Education Circular* 10/65. London: Department of Education and Science, 1965.

13 Central Advisory Council for Education. *Children and Their Primary Schools: The Plowden Report.* London: HMSO, 1967.

14 Royal College of Nursing. *School Nurses: Results from a Census Survey of RCN School Nurses in 2005.* London: Royal College of Nursing, 2005.

15 Secretary of State for Social Services. *The Court Report: Fit for the Future.* London: UK Commission of Enquiry of Child Health Services, 1976.

16 British Paediatric Association. *Report of a Joint Working Party on Health Needs of School Aged Children* (Chaired by Professor Leon Polnay). London: British Paediatric Association, 1995.

17 Kelly A, Mabbett G, Thomé R. Professions and community nursing. In: Symonds A, Kelly A, eds. *The Social Construction of Community Care.* Basingstoke: Macmillan, 1998.

18 United Kingdom Central Council for Nursing, Midwifery and Health Visiting. *The Future of Professional Practice – The Council's Standard for Education and Practice Following Registration.* London: United Kingdom Central Council for Nursing, Midwifery and Health Visiting, 1994.

19 United Kingdom Central Council for Nursing, Midwifery and Health Visiting. *The Code of Professional Conduct.* London: United Kingdom Central Council for Nursing, Midwifery and Health Visiting, 1992.

20 National Leadership and Innovation Agency for Healthcare. Financial help for healthcare students in Wales (available at www.wales.nhs.uk/sites3). Accessed 10 October 2008.

21 Cumberlege J, ed. *Neighbourhood Nursing: A Focus for Care.* London: Department of Health and Social Security, HMSO, 1986.

22 NHS Scotland. *Family Health in Scotland: A Report on the WHO Europe Pilot* (available at www.scotland.gov.uk/publications/2003/10/18428/28397). Edinburgh: Scottish Executive, 2003. Accessed 4 August 2008.

23 Brazier M, Cave E. *Medicine, Patients and the Law,* 4th edn. London: Penguin Books, 2007.

24 Department of Health. *Looking for a School Nurse* (available at www.everychildmatters.gov.uk). Nottingham: Department of Health; Department for Education and Skills, 2006. Accessed November 2006.

25 Department of Health. *Looking for a School Nurse* (available at www.everychildmatters.gov.uk). Nottingham: Department of Health; Department for Education and Skills, 2006, p. 8. Accessed November 2006.

26 Nursing and Midwifery Council. *The Code: Standards of Conduct Performance and Ethics for Nurses and Midwives.* London: Nursing and Midwifery Council, 2008.

27 Griffith R, Tengnah C. *Law and Professional Issues in Nursing (Transforming Nursing Practice Series).* Exeter: Learning Matters, 2008, p. 32.

28 Dimond B. *Legal Aspects of Nursing,* 5th edn. Harlow Essex: Pearson Education Limited, 2008.

29 Tracing Acts of Parliament: House of Commons Information Office. Factsheet L12 (available at http://www.parliament.uk/documents/upload/L12.pdf). Accessed 4 April 2008.

30 Clothier Report. *The Allitt Inquiry: An Independent Inquiry Relating to the Deaths and Injuries on the Children's Ward at Grantham and Kesteven General Hospital during the Period of February to April 1991.* London: HMSO, 1994.

31 United Nations Children's Fund. Convention on the Rights of the Child. General Assembly Resolution 44/25 of 20 November 1989 (available at www.unicef.org/crc/). Accessed 1 September 2008.

32 Beauchamp TL, Childress JF. *Principles of Biomedical Ethics.* Oxford: Oxford University Press, 2001.

33 Department of Health. *Good Practice in Consent: Implementation Guide.* London: Department of Health, 2001.

34 Griffiths R, Tengnah C. *Law and Professional Issues in Nursing* (available at www.learningmatters.co.uk). Exeter: Learning Matters Ltd., 2008.

35 *Re W (a minor: medical treatment)* [1992] 4 All ER 627.

36 Sterrick MJ. Competence in children has a Scottish twist. *BMJ* 2006; **332**: 975.

37 *Gillick v West Norfolk and Wisbech Area Health Authority* [1986] AC 112, [1985] 3 All ER 402, [1985] 2BMLR 11 HL.

38 Department of Health. *Best Practice Guidance for Doctors and Other Health Professionals on the Provision of Advice and Treatment to Young People Under 16 on Contraception, Sexual Health and Reproduction.* Gateway Reference 3382, 2004.

39 Department of Health. *Chief Nursing Officer's Review of the Nursing, Midwifery and Health Visiting Contribution to Vulnerable People and Young People.* London: Department of Health, 2004.

40 Elfer P, Gattis S. Keeping children healthy. In: *Charting Child Health Services.* London: Allen and Unwin National Children's Bureau, 1990, pp. 1-136.

41 Appleton JV. Vulnerable children. In: DeBell D, ed. *Public Health Practice and the School-Age Population.* London: Hodder Arnold, 2007.

42 DeBell D, Everett G. *In a Class Apart: A Study of School Nursing.* Norwich: Norfolk Health Authority, 1997.

43 Baker J, Hallet J, Knox G. *Excluded but not Rejected.* London: The Evangelical Alliance, 1999.

44 United Nations. *Convention on the Rights of the Child.* Article 24 General Assembly resolution 44/25 of 20 November 1989. United Nations Children's Fund (available at www.unicef.org/crc/); 1989.

45 United Nations. *Convention on the Rights of the Child.* Article 24 General Assembly resolution 44/25 of 20 November 1989. United Nations Children's Fund (available at www.unicef.org/crc/), Article 24(2(e); 1989.

46 NHS Litigation Authority. Report of Accounts 2007 (HC 908). London: HMSO, The Stationery Office, 2007.

47 *Donoghue v Stevenson* [1932] AC582.

48 *Bolam v Friern HMC* [1957] 1WLR 582.

49 *Bolitho v City and Hackney Health Authority* [1998] AC 232.

50 *Wilsher v Essex Health Authority* [1988] AC 1074 (HL).

51 *British Home Stores Ltd v Burchell* [1980] ICR 303 (EAT).

52 Nursing and Midwifery Council. *The PREP Handbook.* London: Nursing and Midwifery Council, 2008.

53 *Hefferon v Committee of the UKCC* [1988] Current Law, May 1988. 221.

54 JM Consulting Ltd. *The Regulation of Nurses, Midwives and Health Visitors: Report on a Review of the Nurses, Midwives and Health Visitors Act 1997.* London: JM Consulting Ltd, 1999.

55 NHS Executive. *Modernising Regulation: The New Nursing and Midwifery Council: A Consultation Document.* London: Department of Health, 2000.

56 Nursing and Midwifery Council. *Standards of Proficiency for Specialist Community Public Health Nursing.* London: Nursing and Midwifery Council, 2004.

57 Nursing and Midwifery Council. *Standards of Proficiency for Specialist Community Public Health Nursing.* London: Nursing and Midwifery Council, 2004, Standard 4.

58 Nursing and Midwifery Council. *Standards of Proficiency for Specialist Community Public Health Nursing.* London: Nursing and Midwifery Council, 2004, Section 7.

59 Nursing and Midwifery Council. *Standards to Support Learning and Assessment in Practice.* London: Nursing and Midwifery Council, 2008.

60 *NHS Employers: Agenda for Change* (available at http://www.nhsemployersorg/pay-conditions/agenda-for-change.cfm?frmAlias=/agendaforchange/). Accessed 30 August 2008.

Chapter 6

School Nursing and School Health Practice

Sarah Sherwin and Mary Smith

Learning objectives

After reading this chapter you will be able to:

- Appreciate how policy relating to school health practice translates into reality
- Discuss how the standards for specialist community public health nursing apply to school nursing
- Appreciate some of the challenges and opportunities that exist in promoting the health of the school-aged population

---

Introduction

The changing face of public health care presents many challenges for school nurses and school health services. The role is moving from being a predominantly task-orientated service delivered just by school nurses to one that is a more complex, responsive, proactive model of preventative health involving a range of professionals within a school health team. This new model seeks to identify and address the health and health-related needs not only of individuals but also groups and communities (see Chapter 5 for development and historical overview of school nursing practice). School nurses provide an important link between school-aged children, their families and carers, health and education professionals, social care services, Primary Care Trusts, Children's Trusts, National Health Service (NHS) Trusts and extended services [1]. Although there may be different models of service delivery, school nurses are in a unique and ideal position to plan, implement and evaluate skilled nursing care in order to meet the public health needs of children, young people and the wider school community. In order for children and young people to fulfil their full potential good health is vital and good habits need to be established in childhood to provide a sound basis for lifelong health and well-being [2].

School nursing is cited by Debell and Tomkins [3] as being the only professional group within the NHS whose remit is to focus entirely on meeting the
health needs of school-aged children and young people and their families, yet
it appears to remain a somewhat invisible service. The discussion that will follow is offered as an initial starting point for those working within the remit of
school health, and practitioners are encouraged to engage with this dialogue
and then explore a wider range of literature.

School nurses are required to meet the demands and challenges of promoting and protecting children and young people's health responding to the
plethora of public health legislation, policies, reports and guidance documents
that have been produced over the past few years [4-8]. One of the most influential is that of Every Child Matters [9], which was given legal status in
the form of the Children Act 2004 [10] and applies to all those services and
agencies working with children and young people. Subsequent policy has been
produced for young people entitled Youth Matters [4] in 2005 and a ten-year
strategy 'Aiming High' [11] outlines how to transform facilities and support
for young people exploring issues around positive outcomes, empowerment,
access and quality. There are five identified outcomes aimed at improving
opportunities for all children and young people:

- Be healthy
- Stay safe
- Enjoy and achieve
- Make a positive contribution
- Achieve economic well-being

Activity 6.1

Consider your own individual strengths and limitations relating to the five
outcomes outlined in the Every Child Matters document, then reflect on
your strengths and limitations. Plan how you might develop your own
skills in helping children and young people you work with to achieve the
five outcomes.

Structure of school health teams

School nurses have historically worked as autonomous practitioners, often
working in isolation purely because they are a much smaller group of community nurses. In 2000, Debell and Jackson [12] suggested a framework which
could be adopted to ensure that school health services are able to deliver
services outlined in government policies (Figure 6.1).

Over recent years, in many areas, services have been restructured to include
team leaders, specialist community public health nurses (SCPHNs), school

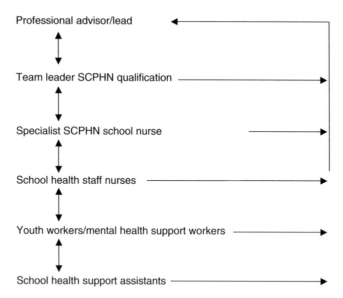

Figure 6.1 Proposed structure of school health team. Adapted from DeBell and Jackson [12].

staff nurses and school nurse support workers. This move towards a multi-skilled school health team, rather than a team of just school nurses has in some areas, helped to provide new, proactive and innovative initiatives designed to improve and protect children's long-term health. The National Service Framework for Children and Young People published in 2004 [6] proposes that school health teams should also include other practitioners such as mental health care workers, youth workers etc. However, the implementation of such a model is fragmented, as there is no national framework for planning and delivering school health services. The number of full-time-qualified school nurses (SCPHNs) have slightly increased [13], but there is still a shortage in meeting the government's commitment of a qualified registered specialist school nurse in every secondary school and its cluster of primary schools in England by 2010 [5]. The Welsh Assembly Government in its policy 'One Wales' [8] also commits to providing a minimum of one family nurse per secondary school.

Nonetheless, the creation of school health teams has started to provide a number of benefits to school nursing. Their conception has helped to reduce the isolation previously felt by some school nurses who have traditionally worked alone managing a caseload [12], as well as introducing a much-needed career structure within the service. Many trusts have been more proactive and invested in employing staff on a variety of different contracts including full-time, all-year-round contracts, which includes school holidays as well contracts that involve evening and weekend working in order to provide a continuous service for children, young people and their families. This coupled with a more flexible working pattern, may help to attract more male, ethnic and other minorities who are currently excluded by the rigidity of limited contracts into school nursing. A team approach is vital, in order for the service to be able to have a robust career structure, which can renew itself, rather than be a stagnant workforce and is designed to meet the need of the school-aged population by including those with the relevant skills.

The development of teams within special schools and the independent sector maybe more problematic due to smaller numbers of children. These particular groups of school nurses tend to deliver more specific and specialised clinical care, supporting children who have long-term conditions or require a more 'first contact' service as in independent schools. Yet, they also have a vital role to play in promoting positive health within the communities that they work with.

Zero- to nineteen-year preventative service

Some services have taken the development of school health teams a stage further and reconfigured to merge health visiting and school nursing services together to provide an integrated 0- to 19-year preventative service in line with integrated children's services and in preparation of delivering the extended Child Health Promotion Programme [14] and Child Health Strategy due to be published in 2009 [15]. A 0- to 19-year preventative service may include SCPHNs, health visitors, occupational health nurses, public health practitioners, youth offending team practitioners, primary mental health workers, youth workers, nursery nurses etc. whoever is required to meet the needs of the population. Such a new way of working has a number of benefits such as providing a more seamless but flexible delivery of services, pooling and local devolvement of budgets and resources to the team and improving the visibility of services working with children and young people. But within such an approach it is important to recognise that specific, specialist skills are still required to meet and respond to the identified needs of children and young people. The 0- to 19-year preventative service would also enable practitioners to extend services to those attending Further Education Colleges and Sixth Form Centres where school health services have traditionally not been provided and by establishing links with occupational health nurses into the workplace where young people may be employed.

Image of school nursing

The image of school nursing is often closely linked to the title 'school nurse' as for some it conjures up historical images of the 'nit nurse'. In an attempt to shake off this old-dated image, a number of services have changed the name, for example, to school health advisors but as this is only at local level this can create confusion for colleagues, children, young people and their families. Some would argue the very title 'school nurse' portrays a very narrow focus of the nurse within the school setting – is it time to change and adopt a title at a national level which reflects the public health role for those aged 0–19 years more closely and that the service should focus on school-aged children and young people wherever they are, not just in schools? Or does the title matter if school nurses are able to market their service, raise their profile and demonstrate the breadth and value of their role? What about the children and young people themselves; what would they prefer the title to be? If they can identify and understand the title then maybe they would be more willing to seek out advice and support.

Specialist community public health nursing and school nursing

Over recent years, school nursing practice has returned to its original remit of promoting and protecting public health focusing on school-aged children, young people and their families (see Chapter 5). It has become increasingly complex and demanding with the need for school nurses to be able to identify, plan, deliver and evaluate health care to meet the needs of the individuals, groups and populations with whom they work. In order to become a registered SCPHN, practitioners must undertake an academic training programme at degree or masters level and meet the standards for SCPHN practice laid down by the Nursing and Midwifery Council [16] which has been discussed in the previous chapter.

These standards are based on four key domains of public health nursing (see Chapter 2). Each of these domains will be explored in more depth in relation to school nursing practice.

Search for health needs

The concept of need is a complex area and open to interpretation; however, Bradshaw [17] identified four types of need: *normative*, *felt*, *expressed* and *comparative* (see Chapters 1 and 2). Any health needs assessment should consider what kind of need is highlighted. Normative need, that is need identified by the health professional, is often used as the basis for health promotion activities. Obtaining views from service users (i.e. teachers, parents and pupils) would help identify felt or expressed needs. Choosing Health [18] highlighted areas of national need including the need to encourage good health by prevention and educational action and to give children and young people a better start in life. School nurses with their knowledge and expertise in health surveillance and health education/promotion are ideally placed to contribute towards programmes to address these needs.

The Children Act 2004 [4] strongly advocates the involvement of children and young people in the planning and delivery of services appropriate to their needs. Involvement of young people from the outset will instil a sense of ownership in initiatives designed to promote health and hopefully will help to ensure that they take on board important messages relating to health and well-being.

Evidence-based practice

There is an assumption that there is little research-based evidence available relating to school nursing practice. However, this view is disputed by DeBell and Tomkins [3], who conducted a comprehensive scoping review of the available evidence. They found that there was a wealth of evidence, but that much of the evidence focuses on individual services rather than painting an overall national picture. This has led to services becoming fragmented nationally and whilst services need to develop to respond to local need, there needs to be a national steering of the profession to establish what is expected from school health services and setting outcome measures. DeBell and Tomkins also identify that there needs to be large-scale research studies into school nurse practice development and school nurse leadership the results of which are needed in order to steer the future direction of the service.

As identified, there is evidence that small-scale studies are taking place and this can contribute to the overall body of school nursing knowledge and be a source of interest and inspiration to others and therefore the findings should also be shared as widely as possible. But the onus is not just on individual practitioners to highlight effective working practices based on research findings. Team leaders, school nurse managers, professional advisors and managers should all play a part in encouraging and actively supporting practitioners to disseminate and publish their work. In support of this concept, Lord Darzi's report [19] on the future direction of the NHS published in 2008, refers to the establishment of a new NHS evidence service where staff will have easy access to clinical and non-clinical best evidence and practice.

Activity 6.2

Reflect on an aspect of your current practice and consider how you know your practice is based on the best evidence available? Spend some time reviewing the current literature to help support, direct and guide your practice.

Health needs assessments and school health plans

The assessment of health needs is a central principle of a public health approach. Assessing the needs of school-aged populations and devising school health plans was advocated back in the early 1990s, but is not a tool that is used universally by school health teams [20]. Health needs assessments aims to help identify, analyse and prioritise the health needs or potential health needs of a population in order to be able to target interventions more appropriately. Assessing need will equip school nurses with essential information relating to the health needs of school-aged children and young people enabling them to prioritise and formulate proactive school health plans. Both schools and school health services are in receipt of a wealth of information that when combined would provide a very clear evidence-based picture of the health needs of that particular group of school-aged children and young people. In turn this would help to inform the provision of health education within the curriculum. School nurses have a considerable working knowledge base relating to the health needs of the local area such as the incidence of dental caries, obesity levels, teenage pregnancy rates, admissions to local accident and emergency departments detailing alcohol and drug misuse, the nature of accidents relating to those that occur within the home or out in the community as well as being cognisant about the availability of local services.

School nurse's knowledge regarding the state of children and young people's health and their ability to build relationships with them and their parents is, according to Debell and Tomkins [3], highly prized. They are often aware of the children's and young people's emotional needs and risk-taking behaviours via the drop in clinics run in many schools. Therefore, it is imperative that schools and health professionals work together seamlessly, combining information and resources in order to plan and deliver a relevant health curriculum. The document 'Looking for a School Nurse' [21] should assist head teachers and governors, both in state and independent schools, to help them work with school nursing services to promote and improve the health of children and young people, as well as staff, within their school community.

This information should be disseminated and used to strategically plan and provide health promotion and public health services in partnership with schools. It should also contribute to local health targets identified by Primary Care Trusts and commissioners and assist in delivering local multi-agency children's and young people's plans. This will involve collaborative working and the development of healthy alliances within education, social care and other agencies working with children, which in turn will raise awareness of the school nurse's role, but most importantly meet the needs of the children and young people.

Case Study 6.1 Searching for health needs: anger management

School health advisors within a West Midlands Primary Care Trust identified a health need in relation to a gap in service provision, for those children and young people who were having difficulty controlling their anger.

The school health advisors contacted the child and family psychology department for assistance in bridging this gap.

A group consisting of a psychologist, a psychology trainer and two school health advisors was formed to develop a project in order to meet this identified need.

A ten-week course was designed based on the cognitive behaviour therapy approach to anger management, utilising best evidence-based practice.

The programme is delivered within schools by school health advisors supported by members from the psychology team. An extensive evaluation of the course is currently in progress and initial indications suggest there has been improvement in the children's behaviour.

Case Study 6.2 Searching for health needs youth advisory clinics

The school nursing team in an area in Wales was aware that only a small number of young people were attending the existing youth advisory clinics (YAS) for sexual health advice, contraceptive services and healthy lifestyles advice.

Using the personal social and health education sessions in schools the team opened a direct route to the YAS clinic. These clinics are run by the school nursing team who has established contacts with young people with a reputation of being trustworthy and approachable.

Since identification of this gap in service provision the number of young people attending YAS clinics has increased considerably.

The venue is young person friendly, confidential and staffed with people trained to work in this area.

However, searching for health needs and delivering services to meet such a need is not without its challenges. An equitable system of health care is one in which everyone has equal opportunities to achieve their potential health status. Bagnall and Dilloway [22] argue that the school health service is able to prevent ill health and promote positive health is an excellent example of a service that is able to put the health of the whole population on an equal basis. However, the diversity in the organisation of school health services, clinical practice and the wide variations in caseload sizes have contributed to an inequitable provision of services nationally.

Facilitating health-enhancing activities

School nurses, along with other agencies, play a major role in facilitating health-enhancing activities for the school-aged population [23]. Involvement in local health promotion programmes as well as embracing national initiatives such as the Healthy Schools Programme all help to enhance children and young people's health. The use of the spiral curriculum to revisit and reinforce health messages is vital, as is the need to work in partnership with the whole school community. Selective health interviews as advocated by Hall and Elliman [24], and drop in sessions provide an arena for individuals to seek confidential advice and information on a variety of health matters. Children and young people are very impressionable and the whole ethos of the health-promoting school can be used to portray positive role models and encourage participation in a huge range of health-enhancing activities.

School health teams are involved in promoting and protecting health in many areas such as running smoking cessation groups, delivering parenting programmes, advising on behavioural issues, delivering immunisation programmes, providing drug and alcohol education etc. The Darzi Review of the NHS [19] reaffirms that there must be comprehensive well-being and prevention services which need to focus on key goals which include tackling childhood obesity and encouraging physical activity, improving sexual health, promoting positive mental health and supporting the vulnerable in society. These key areas will be discussed in more depth.

Childhood obesity

Childhood obesity in the UK has increased dramatically over recent years and there is increasing concern about the effects on children's long-term health [25]. The causes of which are multi-factorial but are largely attributed to the increase in availability of high energy, low nutritional, cheap foods high in fat, sugar and salt as well as high sugary fizzy drinks. Combined with the downward trend in physical exercise, due to the use of small-screen games consoles, mobile phones, televisions and computers and the fact that children have more limited opportunities for play, have all played a part in the obesity revolution [26]. Not only does this have implications for the child or young person in terms of their short- and long-term physical and mental health, that can affect their educational and employment attainment but also has a significant impact on the NHS [27].

The Foresight report [28] is a report commissioned by the government to develop a long-term vision over the next 40 years to reduce obesity levels within the UK. The report stated that by 2050, 60% of men and 50% of women will be obese at a cost of £45 billion pounds if no action is taken. There is a strong correlation between children becoming obese if one or both parents are obese. In boys this is around 25% and in girls around 22%.

It has taken 30 years for obesity trends to have developed and changes will not occur overnight. The report advocates that for obesity levels to be halted it will require partnership working between government, science, business and civil society and at multiple levels personal, family, community and national. It is recognised that the causes of obesity are multi-factorial and include diet, access to reasonably priced healthy foods, the need for safe environments and communities so children can play safely, access to sport and leisure facilities, social marketing, healthy schools and workplaces etc. But these all are issues that a school nurse who has been trained as a SCPHN (supported by other members of the school health team) can help to address.

> **Activity 6.3**
>
> Considering the important role parents play in their child's nutrition, reflect on what level of support and type of advice you give to parents/carers.
>
> How can you further support families to make behavioural changes in relation to their child and family's nutrition? Consider the strategies and initiatives you and your team could be involved in to promote good nutrition practices with children, parents and carers?
>
> How can you promote the Change4Life Programme with parents and children? (www.dh.gov.uk/change4life)

Tackling childhood obesity is a national priority for the NHS and local partners, and is part of the government's new public service agreement (PSA) on child health and well-being. Following evidence provided by the Foresight report, a cross-government strategy, *Healthy Weight: Healthy Lives*, published by the Department of Health in 2008 [27, p. 7] sets out the following target:

> Our ambition is to be the first major nation to reverse the rising tide of obesity and overweight in the population by ensuring that everyone is able to achieve and maintain a healthy weight. Our initial focus will be on children, by 2020 we aim to reduce the proportion of overweight and obese children to 2000 levels.

Box 6.1 shows the government's areas for tackling obesity and excess weight in children.

> **Box 6.1   Five areas for tackling excess weight (*Healthy Weight: Healthy Lives: A Cross Government Strategy*) [27]**
>
> **Children: healthy growth and healthy weight** – early prevention of weight problems to avoid the 'conveyor-belt' effect into adulthood
>
> **Promoting healthier food choices** – reducing the consumption of foods that are high in fat, sugar and salt and increasing the consumption of fruit and vegetables
>
> **Building physical activity into our lives** – getting people moving as a normal part of their day
>
> **Creating incentives for better health** – increasing the understanding and value people place on the long-term impact of decisions
>
> **Personalised advice and support** – complementing preventative care with treatment for those who already have weight problems

Activity 6.4

Consider the five main themes outlined in the document 'Healthy Weight: Healthy Lives' (www.dh.gov.uk/healthyweighthealthylives).
Consider how school nurses and school health teams can deliver and evaluate these themes within practice.

Physical activity

Play and physical activity play a crucial role in a child's development. It helps the child to develop physical control as well as gross and fine motor coordination. It also plays an important role in promoting good health and preventing and tackling childhood obesity.

Encouraging regular exercise has been a key element of a number of government policies over the past few years for both adults as well as children and young people. School health teams are able to promote and support children, young people and their families to engage in physical activity by running 'fit clubs' outside of school curriculum or being involved in weight management programmes that have a fitness element.

Case Study 6.3 Facilitating health-enhancing activities: physical exercise sessions for children

School nurses within an area of the West Midlands have a specialist team called Phyzkids, which provides physical activity sessions for children aged 5-12 years. The team is made up of approximately ten school nurses with three of them having undergone specialist training (Fitkid) in order to lead the sessions. Each session lasts for approximately one hour with 4-5 fun activities, including warm-up, cool-down and circle-time. Activities are designed to be adaptable for varying abilities to ensure all children can be included. There are six progressive sessions, which have imaginative themes, for example, in the army, seaside fun, grab five and bone builders. As well as encouraging physical activity and why it is important for good health the sessions are also designed to incorporate other health promotion messages, for example healthy eating and sun safety.

Mental health

School health teams need to provide holistic care to children and young people so they can develop into healthy adults and have the ability to develop psychologically, emotionally, intellectually and spiritually. Children's and young people's social and emotional well-being is important as it affects their physical health and determines what they achieve at school and whether they can choose to adopt a healthy lifestyle. The National Institute for Health and Clinical Excellence (NICE) [29] have produced guidance for promoting children's social and emotional well-being in primary education. A stark message is that a lack of investment in mental health promotion in primary schools is likely to lead to a significant cost for future generations.

Prevalence of mental health disorders in school-aged children

Statistics from the Office of National Statistics [30] suggest that 1:10 children aged between 5 and 16 years have a diagnosable mental health disorder. It is estimated that between 1:12 and 1:15 children self-harm and 25 000 children are serious enough to admit to hospital and for children who are in the 'looked after' system this is much higher, school nurses have seen a rise in children suffering from stress and anxiety; 1:10 children have a mental health problem, that is serious enough to seek professional help [31]. The impact of transition periods plays a role in affecting mental health such as changing schools, illness, family divorce, bereavement and loss and those separated from their families for a variety of reasons. For these reasons children need to develop coping mechanisms to cope with such changes and school nursing services need to reflect this; by providing initiatives that will enhance every aspect of their childhood.

Role of school health teams in promoting positive mental health

School nurses are able to help deliver emotional health and well-being programmes as part of a school's curriculum, can support individual children and young people by providing early intervention services, and provide intensive support to children, young people and their families around transition periods. School nurses can work with schools to run bullying support groups for both the bullied child as well as the perpetrator. Signposting to other services such as child and adolescent mental health, bereavement services, peer support groups etc. is also an important aspect of the role. However, many services find it difficult to provide such services due to workforce numbers and the need for commissioners to recognise the importance of investing in more school nurses to meet this important health need. There are some services which have a school nurse specialising in emotional health and well-being and mental health or employ specialist mental health workers within the team to support children and young people. There are a number of examples across the country where pupils are being supported in relation to emotional health such as the one detailed below.

> **Case Study 6.4** Facilitation of health-enhancing activities: stress management programme run by school nurses
>
> An aromatherapy service has been set up in local high school, within the West Midlands, by a school nurse, who is also a qualified complementary therapist, to help reduce stress and anxiety in young people. They may be experiencing difficulties due to family breakdowns, loss, illnesses and exam pressures. The treatment is based on hand massage and relaxation techniques. This initiative has been successful because of support from the PCT and the school. Funding has been obtained from the Community Partnership Fund and set up at a minimal cost. The young people can self-refer or are referred by agencies such as Child and Adolescent Mental Health Services and teachers within the school community. The evaluations of the service have been very positive and the aim is to develop and extend the service to other local schools in the near future.

Sexual health

It is acknowledged that the UK has the highest teenage conception rates within Western Europe [32] and it appears unlikely that the target to reduce under-18 conception rates by 2010, as stated in Choosing Health [5], will be met. The Social Exclusion Unit Report on Teenage Pregnancy in 1999 [32] identified that there was no one single reason for the high rates but highlighted three factors that appear to contribute – low expectations of young people many from disadvantaged backgrounds, ignorance about the need for contraception and its availability, sexually transmitted infections and the demands of parenting and mixed messages that as a society we portray to our young people about sex. In 66% of teenage pregnancies there is a live full-term birth and it is recognised that teenage parents are then more likely to experience long-term unemployment, have less educational opportunities, live in inadequate housing all of which contribute to health, social and economic inequalities [32, 33].

School nurses involved in working with young people need to be trained in order to deliver effective sex and relationship education both with groups and individuals. It may be pertinent for services to consider employing, as part of the school health team, school nurses that specialise in adolescent health. It is important that it is not only knowledge and information that is communicated but young people need to be able to develop skills and attitudes to make informed, safe choices that will protect their long-term health. (This will be discussed later in this chapter.) Chlamydia screening, pregnancy testing etc. can all be offered at drop-in clinics but often this is reliant on the views of the head teacher, school governors and ethos of the school.

School nurses need to work closely with schools and other agencies to over-come some of these challenges particularly in areas where teenage conception rates and sexually transmitted infections are high.

Supporting children and young people with complex health needs

Children and young people with complex needs also require high levels of sup-port by school health services and partner agencies [34]. Over recent years there has been a significant move to educate children with complex needs in mainstream school partly in response to the Special Educational Needs Disability Act 2001 [35]. The number of children with special needs or com-plex health needs attending mainstream schools has gradually increased over the years with an estimated 2.8% of all children having a statement of spe-cial educational needs [36]. There are, of course, many more children within mainstream schools who, despite having some form of special needs, do not require a statement. This widespread integration has resulted in a changing role within special schools, as only 36.9% of children with a statement of special educational needs actually attended a special school.

School nurses in special schools are required to care for children with very complex health needs, but school nurses working in mainstream schools tend to have less input for the day-to-day care (as this is often carried out by support staff who is with the child all day in school). The generic school nurse is more involved in drawing up plans of care that support the child, parents and school, bringing together agencies to ensure the needs of the child are met. School nurses not only have a role to play in the assessment procedure but also with 'inclusiveness' comes the need to acquire knowledge and understanding of a wide range of conditions. In order to facilitate effective integration, school nurses should understand the effect these conditions may have on a child's ability to learn, thus enabling them to offer advice and support to the child, family and school staff. The Children's Plan [37] highlights the importance of providing ongoing support to young people and their families during the transition from children's to adult services.

Case Study 6.5 Facilitation of health-enhancing activities: obesity

Poor nutrition in the South Wales Valleys has been a longstanding prob-lem with obesity identified as a major issue throughout Wales.

The school nursing team addressed this need by providing nutrition-based activities in the schools in a phased and age-related manner as part of the school curriculum.

An innovative interactive Treasure Island Game was implemented to help raise awareness of food groups and enable primary school chil-dren to make healthier food choices and is well received by schools and children.

> Additional activities include healthy pack lunches, hydration awareness and food advertising. These health promotion activities enable individual schools to work towards achieving the national-recognised healthy school's award.

Personal, social and health education

Personal, social and health education (PSHE), although not a statutory curriculum subject, is delivered in most schools and is one of the four key themes outlined in the Healthy Schools Programme. The PSHE Continuing Professional Development programme is a national scheme that has been developed for teachers, community nurses and other professionals who work both in schools and out in the community. The need for the development of specialist teams to be established, particularly within secondary schools, which consists of specialist trained teachers and other health professionals such as school nurses and sexual health nurse advisors was recommended as being a way forward by OFSTED in 2002 [38].

The programme aims to:

- Improve the confidence of teachers, community nurses and others delivering PSHE in schools and out of schools settings
- Provide recognition for individual teachers' and community nurses' experience and skills
- Improve the quality and effectiveness of PSHE provided to children and young people
- Raise the profile of PSHE
- Contribute to the United Kingdom's teenage pregnancy strategy's goal to halve the number of under-18 conception rates by 2010 [32]
- Address issues relating to health inequalities and social inclusion

This programme is an effective example of a joint approach between different government departments and provides clear leadership between services that is able to transfer policy into practice [3].

The programme also enables schools, communities and their health partners to take a more strategic, coherent approach to PSHE, as the priority that is given to PSHE within a school can often depend on the interest and motivation of individual teachers and community nurses that happen to be working in the area.

In some schools, where PSHE is not given priority, it maybe the view of the head teacher and governing body that it should be the parents and carers who should play the major role in meeting the personal, social and health needs of their children rather than the school itself. The opposite may also be true in that some parents rely solely on the school to inform their children about health particularly in relation to puberty and Sexual relationship education (SRE). But what remains clear is that children and young people need to be given every opportunity to develop knowledge, skills and attitudes to enable them to make informed health choices.

> **Case Study 6.6** School nurse's experience of PSHE programme
>
> 'Before undertaking the PSHE programme I just went into school and delivered information on health. Completing the course has enabled me to consider the importance of planning sessions in conjunction with the teacher to ensure the session actually meets the needs of the whole group as well as evaluating the effectiveness of the session with the pupils. I now feel much more confident in delivering PSHE'.

Promoting health outside of the school curriculum

It is recognised that schools play a vital role and are a key setting in order to promote health [5, 39], but do not have the monopoly on promoting children's and young people's health. School-based health promotion is only one influence on the health behaviour of young people [40] as schools are not the only place where children and young people gather. Children and young people gather in a whole host of other settings, which can contribute in supporting them to make well-chosen health choices such as youth centres. Learning is ongoing and takes place outside of the school environment in the home, from television, via the Internet and in the wider community. All of these will influence children's and young people's beliefs about health and illness. Health promotion programmes can and should also be delivered outside of the normal school curriculum in a variety of other settings where young people gather such as youth clubs and groups, sports clubs, support groups, children's centres, activities and groups run with extended schools, breakfast clubs, after-school clubs, young peoples' sexual health clinics, Sure Start Plus programmes, Flying Start in Wales, young offenders institutions in fact anywhere where children and young people come together.

The issue of access to a health service designed for school-aged children and young people must also be considered for those who do not regularly attend mainstream school. This may be for a variety of reasons such as chronic illness, home-educated, behaviour problems, pregnancy, teenage mothers, young carers etc. It is recognised that those not attending school maybe potentially more vulnerable from developing long-term health problems [32]. They require equal access, alongside their peers who attend mainstream school, to a health care professional who is specifically trained to work with school-aged children and young people. Research carried out by Lightfoot and Bines in 1997 [41] suggests that whilst school nurses are well placed to meet the health needs of children and young people within the school setting, young people value a choice in being able to access similar services outside of the school premises. New models of service delivery, such as integrated teams with specialist nurses, that are both creative and innovative, need to be developed to ascertain how school health services can effectively meet the health needs of children and young people (up to the age of 19 years) wherever they are.

School health teams have the skills to be able to meet the health needs of school-aged children and young people wherever they are, what is required is additional resources and an increase in workforce capacity. This reinforces the public health role of the school nurse, recognising that the role stretches beyond the confines of the school and into the wider community. In order for this to take place effectively, school nurses need to work closely with other agencies from both the statutory and voluntary sectors to create opportunities for the promotion and development of health promoting initiatives, which meet the health, needs of the children and young people they are working with. However, this can only happen if there is long-term sustainable investment in the school health service.

> ## Activity 6.5
>
> Consider your role or your team's role in supporting children and young people outside of the school setting. Justify your involvement and consider how you could provide evidence to commissioners of your/your team's effectiveness.

Stimulating an awareness of health needs

Health education and health promotion are essential factors in raising awareness amongst the school community. The Healthy Schools Programme which was re-launched in 2005, aims to raise awareness of the opportunities that exist in schools for improving health and develop a whole school approach to health around four core themes of healthy eating, PSHE, emotional health and well-being and physical activity [42]. A National Healthy Schools Network and the Wired for Health website support the initiative, which is not only concerned with promoting pupils' health but includes the whole school community.

Consulting children, young people and parents in relation to health issues

In order to stimulate effectively an awareness of health needs it is important to consult and work with users of the service.

In the early years of the education system and within society children were viewed as passive recipients of knowledge and information. Mayall [43] makes the point that children did not speak for themselves but were spoken for by adults. They construct their understandings about what children need and decisions are made which is the basis on which children lead their lives. But the introduction of the United Nations Convention for the Rights of the Child Articles 12, 13 and 17 brought the entitlement of children and young people to participate to the fore [44].

There has been a conscious move to move away from the traditional paternalistic style of service delivery to one that should encourage children and young people to actively participate in their own health care agenda [5]. Young people define health holistically and have a good understanding of what is considered to be healthy and unhealthy. However, it is the environment and their lifestyle that does not always help them to choose healthy options [45].

One of the principles of the Children's Plan [46] is that services need to be shaped and developed by children, young people and their families not designed around professional boundaries. The Chief Nursing Review in 2004 [47] highlighted that children and young people wanted services that listened to them, were accessible, confidential, non-judgemental and provided information that was age appropriate in order for them to make choices. Children with disabilities also wanted to be given information and choices about their care and treatment. The Department of Health has developed quality criteria titled 'You're Welcome' [48] that provides guidance on how to make health services young people friendly.

An initial step is to consult the views of those who use the service, which not only include the children but the views of the parents and wider school community. On a school community basis the views of young people may be sought via student councils which exist in many secondary schools and increasingly so in junior schools. OFSTED in 2002 [38] found that few schools engaged pupils in planning or evaluating sex and relationship education programmes or policies. However, they highlighted that in some areas consultations do take place and where this occurs pupils value such discussions and the school gains fresh insights into their curriculum, which assists in future development. The Education Act 2002 [49] requires that all schools include pupils in the decision-making processes relating to issues within school life that affect them. Schools need to consult children and young people and respond to their needs to ensure that PSHE is relevant, effective and that the potential for learning is maximised fully [50].

Accessing existing research studies such as lifestyle surveys and conducting local research projects are also ways of seeking the views regarding health of the 'whole population' within the school. School health assessments and the establishment of service-level agreements are also ideal opportunities to seek the views of teaching staff, school governors as well as the children. Involving parents in clinical audits and 'customer satisfaction' surveys as well as attendance at parents' evenings are additional mechanisms. Although the users of the service maybe consulted and have some control over the delivery of existing services, they should equally be consulted and actively involved in identifying and planning new services. For example, if a new drop-in clinic is to be set up then it is important to have representation from the young people who will be accessing the clinic. In some areas young people are being included in recruitment processes for school health staff either meeting candidates informally before the interview or as part of the interviewing process itself. There does, however, need to be a conscious effort to ensure this does not become an example of notional empowerment. A more committed approach to truly empowering young people in decision-making processes is to have a representative from this group on working parties and steering groups. Emphasis must be placed on consultation, participation and responding to expressed needs rather than just monitoring and recording opinions which are then largely ignored. Although there needs to be a recognition that there are often only limited resources available, but school health service managers need to be creative with the funds that are available and seek further investment on a number of different levels – micro (Primary Care Trusts, NHS Trusts in Wales), meso (Children Trusts and Strategic Health Authorities) and macro (Government and European sources).

Acting as an advocate for school-aged children

School nurses are ideally placed to act as advocates for the school-aged children and young people. For example in situations where there are issues related to safeguarding such as abuse, witnessing domestic abuse, bullying, experiencing bereavement or loss or where there is low self esteem.

Indeed client or patient advocacy is an integral and essential aspect of good professional practice, and is implicit within the code: standards of conduct, performance and ethics for nurses and midwives [51]. Therefore, school nurses have a duty to act as advocates for school-aged children.

Providing support to parents, in partnership with other agencies, can be an important role for school nurses. This can be in the form of parenting support groups for both primary- and secondary-aged children, behaviour management groups, individual support at family level etc.

The notion of providing personalised care is revisited in the Darzi report on the NHS [19]. Such an approach will help and support people of all ages including children and young people to stay healthy and protect their long-term health. One example of this is the NHS Teen LifeCheck initiative, which is an online self-assessment tool for 11-14 year old. Its aim is to provide information and advice on healthy lifestyle issues and signpost young people to further sources of advice at both a local and national level [52].

Collaborative working

One of the key principles of the modernised primary care-led NHS is collaboration and partnership working [18]. Working alongside other agencies has been a central feature of the school health service, as it owes its very existence to working with education providers, working with social workers to safeguard children and young people and with other agencies such as CAMHS, police etc. Many school nurses run drop-in clinics in conjunction with youth workers, educational welfare officers, community paediatricians, dieticians etc. and need to develop clear links with general practice [53]. But possibly this could be described as working in parallel rather than true partnership working [23]. There have been challenges over the years as school health services have only been able to work in schools by invitation. Often social workers, education staff and school health have all been working with a child and their family with little communication taking place between them. Every Child Matters [7] seeks to address some of these shortcomings. However, the Children Act 2004 [54] has provided a legislative framework to ensure these processes become formalised with a plethora of supporting documentation to aid schools, health services, social care and other key partners in the establishment of Children's Trust.

Children's Trusts will support the development of initiatives such as extended schools. There is no 'blueprint' of what an extended school must look like as it should be tailor made to meet the needs of the local community and reflect its diversity [55] but it may also strengthen services already currently provided. Fundamental to the development of extended services is the consultation and involvement of the wider community. The idea of bringing services together is to make it easier for universal services (such as schools) to work with specialist and targeted services such as school health [56].

During recent years there has been other commitments to facilitate a greater understanding of the importance of working together to improve services for children and young people. At a local level Children and Young People's Services Delivery Plans have been developed by all those agencies involved in delivering children's services and this should also foster a commitment in providing joined-up integrated seamless services.

Interprofessional learning is now a key feature of many specialist community public health nursing courses with community nurses learning alongside social workers and police officers, for example. Other educational programmes such as the National PSHE CPD Programme enables teachers and community nurses to learn and work together.

Case Study 6.7 Interprofessional collaboration placement project between trainee teachers and school nurses

Seven trainee teachers and eight student school nurses took part in a joint placement project within a secondary school in the West Midlands, facilitated by lecturers from the University of Wolverhampton. The aim of the project was to bring together teachers and school nurses to work together to plan, deliver and evaluate a PSHE day for pupils ranging from year 6 to year 13 and to promote a greater understanding of each other's roles in relation to meeting the five outcomes outlined in Every Child Matters.

The teachers were able to share their knowledge and skills around lesson planning and classroom management and the school nurses were able to provide information on health issues and resources that could be utilised. In conjunction with the school a range of appropriate topics were identified and the group worked in pairs to plan a PSHE lesson.

The students as well as school staff and pupils evaluated the lessons and the school reported that 'this was the most successful PSHE day they have held'. It is anticipated that this project will be offered to other schools within the area.

Influencing policy development

The contribution school nurses make to the assessment of health needs and the promotion and protection of health places them in a prime position to influence and contribute to the development of effective health policies. In broad terms, there is also a role for acting as an advocate for school communities, in relation to policy formulation on health issues. It is, however, recognised that there needs to be opportunities available for children and young people to be able to verbalise their opinions, thoughts and ideas [41]. School nurses (in conjunction with other colleagues from education and youth services) are in a position to be able to facilitate these opportunities and communicate them to those involved in policy formulation and the planning of health care services.

Ways of being involved in developing policy

Being involved in policy development can be achieved in several ways; at school level, school nurses can contribute to the Healthy Schools Programme [42] by acting as a facilitator working with school staff, governors, parents and pupils, assisting schools to develop bullying and SRE policies, for example. At a community level school nurses are able to adopt a strategic stance working in partnership with other agencies in order to plant the needs of school-aged children firmly on the health, education and social care agenda. For this to be maximised school nurses need to have representation at a strategic level within Primary Care Trusts, NHS Trusts, Children's Trusts, Strategic Health Authorities and Local Authorities/Extended Services Provision. Influence at national level can be achieved by becoming actively involved in professional organisations, contributing to government consultations, presenting at conferences, publishing, getting involved in and undertaking research and lobbying for change.

Case Study 6.8 How school nurses have contributed to the development of the immunisation policy for a Midlands Primary Care Trust

'As part of our Specialist Community Public Health Nurse (SCPHN) degree we were given the opportunity to work in partnership with the PCT's Immunisation Officer. We contributed comprehensively towards the development of the new immunisation policy for use by staff working within the Primary Care Trust.

Using information gained from policy development discussions on the SCPHN course we felt confident in using our analytical skills and knowledge to participate in detailed discussions on contentious issues such as consent. An initial draft was prepared and following further appraisal this was amended, as it was agreed aspects of the policy were difficult to understand. The vaccination and immunisation committee will now review the final draft of the policy.

Our involvement in the development of the policy was a new and exciting challenge and something that we would not have felt confident in doing before undertaking the SCPHN course'.

Activity 6.6

Reflect on how you have worked with another agency and consider the factors that made the experience successful or not. List the things you would do next time to improve the partnership and collaboration and ultimately improve the health outcomes for the child, young person and their family.

Summary

Chapters 5 and 6 have provided an overview of some of the many, complex issues related to school health practice. It was not possible, nor intended, to provide in-depth analysis of the areas rather to stimulate thoughts and motivate school nurses and those working in school health teams to seek further information. School nursing has changed considerably since its inception over a hundred years ago, although the principles remain similar. The government has acknowledged the valuable contribution that school nurses can make to the public health agenda [6–8]. School nurses, school health teams and 0–19 years' preventative services continue to work hard to raise the profile of their profession and prove their worth as key specialists working to improve the health of children and young people in schools, colleges and in other settings.

The demands on school health services are ever growing both nationally and at a local level. School nurses have hungered for national recognition to demonstrate that they are able to effectively identify and contribute to meeting the health needs of Britain's school-aged children. A plethora of government policies has supported this recognition, but the service needs to continue to respond to the challenge of ensuing that there is a firm structure in place, which will meet these ever-increasing demands, for example the introduction of the HPV vaccine for protection against cervical cancer [57]. Whilst this is clearly a public health issue that school health teams are ideally placed to deliver on, the resource implications are huge and the service has currently not got sufficient capacity to absorb this new initiative, and if they do it will be at the demise of some other very important aspect of the role. Therefore, it is important that new programmes and initiatives such as the proposed extension to the Child Health Promotion Programme [37] are adequately centrally funded, and that recognition is given to school health services that they can with the right resources implement and manage these public health initiatives.

School nurses must be prepared to engage in research, share areas of innovation and good practice by the publication of articles, projects, disseminating at conferences in order to establish a clear-evidence base and expand the body of school nursing knowledge. Although school nurses are involved in very valuable work, the service needs to be able to demonstrate that its outcomes are clinically effective and that there is a commitment to strive to continuously improve the quality of the service provided. The continued introduction of commissioning will influence the direction of community nursing service including school nursing. The Darzi report [19] clearly highlights that community nurses will have a role to play in the commissioning process. School nurses and their managers are in a position to advise on and influence the development and commissioning of services in relation to children's and young people's health.

However, whilst adopting a strategic approach in developing closer links with primary care is essential equilaterally, school nursing services need to be able to demonstrate to commissioners, through evidence-based practice that the service provided actually meets the health needs of school communities [53, 3]. There needs to be clear evidence that a wide range of strategies and clinically audited interventions (which have a public health focus) are in place and are clinically effective. Whilst strategic players such as team leaders, professional advisors, managers, commissioners and providers have responsibility for such developments, it is ultimately the responsibility of every school nurse to seek out the health needs of children and young people.

Consideration also needs to be given to marketing and recruitment. As a multi-cultural society deliberation must be given to the needs of all groups and as such school health services should continue to strive to attract nurses from different ethnic groups, to increase the number of male nurses within the profession and provide a structured career pathway to encourage newly qualified staff.

The title 'school nurse' needs to be debated in order to ensure that it accurately reflects the modern role and in the light of new models of service delivery. Another important area to be addressed is related to contracted working hours, there must be adequate numbers of school nurses and support staff working full-time in order to provide a continuous, seamless service for children and young adults throughout the year both in schools and in other settings. In areas where school nurses work on a term-time basis parents and young people may feel isolated during school holidays at a time when they also lose the support of the school environment.

School health teams need good leadership from within, working at a strategic level in partnership with others locally and nationally, to develop cost-effective services, which prove the true value of investing in services for school-aged children and young people.

The diverse nature of current school nursing practice will strongly influence the opportunities that exist for developing relationships within primary care. However, in an NHS that is largely primary care led and in the new world of commissioning services, it is essential for school nurses and school health to be able to respond to the challenge of creating a new service agenda, by reducing the invisibility of the service, being responsive and proactive. This chapter has identified just a few of the many examples across the country where school nurses are working in new ways, but these need to be adopted at a more national level, with the flexibility to ensure the specific health needs of local school-aged populations are still met. It will take a firm commitment to continue to develop a truly integrated approach in promoting the public health of school-aged children and young people within local schools, colleges and the wider community. We owe it to the future health of the next adult generation, to promote and protect their health, which is one of the most fundamental principles of school health practice. However, there must be an inspired shared vision at a local and national strategic level in order for the profession to continue on the challenging but exciting journey translating rhetoric into reality.

References

1 DeBell D, Everett G. The changing role of school nursing with health education and health promotion. *Health Education* 1998; **98**(3): 107-15.
2 Department for Children, Schools and Families. *The Children's Plan: Building Brighter Futures* (available at www.dcsf.gov.uk). London: TSO, 2007. Accessed 6 August 2008.
3 Debell D, Tomkins A. *Discovering the Future of School Nursing: The Evidence Base*. London: CPHVA, 2006.
4 *Children Act* (available at www.publications.parliament.uk); 2004. Accessed 30 April 2008.

5 Department of Health. *Choosing Health: Making Healthier Choices Easier.* London: The Stationery Office, 2004.

6 Department of Health. *National Service Framework for Children, Young People and Maternity Services.* London: TSO, 2004.

7 Department for Education and Skills (DfES)/Department of Health (DH). *Every Child Matters: Change for Children.* London: HMSO, The Stationery Office, 2004.

8 Welsh Assembly Government. *One Wales: A Progressive Agenda for the Government of Wales.* Cardiff: WAG, 2007.

9 Department for Education and Skills (DfES)/Department of Health (DH). *Every Child Matters.* London: TSO, 2003.

10 Department of Children, Schools and Families. *Youth Matters.* London: TSO, 2005.

11 Department of Children, Schools and Families. *Aiming High for Young People: Ten Year Strategy for Positive Outcomes* (available at www.hm-treasury. gov.uk). London: DCSF/HM Treasury, 2007. Accessed 9 October 2008.

12 DeBell D, Jackson P. *School Nursing within the Public Health Agenda: A Strategy for Practice.* London: QNI, 2000.

13 CPHVA. *Community Practitioner, Editorial.* 2008; **81**(5): 4.

14 Department of Health. *Pregnancy and the First Five Years of Life.* London: TSO, 2007.

15 Department for Children, Schools and Families. *The Children's Plan: Building Brighter Futures* (available at www.dcsf.gov.uk). London: TSO, 2007. Accessed 10 October 2008.

16 Nursing and Midwifery Council. *Standards of Proficiency for Specialist Community Public Health Nurses* (available at www.nmc-uk.org). London: Nursing and Midwifery Council, 2004.

17 Bradshaw J. The concept of social need. *New Society* 1972; **19**: 640-43.

18 Department for Health. *Choosing Health: Making Healthier Choices Easier.* London: The Stationery Office, 2004.

19 Department of Health. *High Quality for All. NHS Next Stage Review: The Darzi Report.* London: TSO, 2008.

20 Royal College of Nursing. *School Profiling.* London: RCN, 1992.

21 Department of Health. *Looking for a School Nurse.* London: DH, 2006.

22 Bagnall P, Dilloway M. *In a Different Light: School Nurses and Their Role in Meeting the Needs of School Age Children.* London: Department of Health, 1996.

23 Sherwin S, Williams A. Promoting health: historical overview and political context. In: Thurtle V, Wright J, eds. *Promoting the Health of School Age Children.* London: Quay Books, 2008.

24 Hall D, Elliman D, eds. *Health for All Children*, Revised 4th edn. Oxford: Oxford University Press, 2006.

25 Foresight report (available at www.foresight.gov.uk); 2007. Accessed 5 August 2008.

26 Office for National Statistics. *National Diet and Nutrition Survey: Young People Aged Four to Eighteen Years. Vol. 1: Report of the Diet and Nutrition Survey.* London: TSO, 2000.

27 Department of Health. *Healthy Weight: Healthy Lives: A Cross Government Strategy for England.* London: TSO, 2008.

28 Foresight report (available at www.foresight.gov.uk); 2007. Accessed 12 September 2008.

29 NICE. *Promoting Children's Social and Emotional Wellbeing in Primary Education. NICE Public Health Guidance 12* (available at www.nice.org.uk). London: NICE, 2008.

30 Office for National Statistics (ONS). *Census 2001 National Report for England and Wales.* London: ONS, 2004.

31 Department for Education and Skills/Department for Health. *School Nurse: Practice Development Resource Pack.* London: DfES Publications, 2006.

32 Social Exclusion Unit (SEU). *Teenage Pregnancy Strategy.* London: SEU, 1999.

33 Department of Health. *Drinking, Smoking and Drug Use in Young People in 2003.* London: HMSO, 2004.

34 *Children Act.* London: HMSO, 1989.

35 *Special Educational Needs Disability Act* (available at www.opsi.gov.uk); 2001. Accessed 1 August 2008.

36 Department for Children, Schools and Families. *Special Educational Needs in England* (available at SFR 15/2008 www.dcsf.gov.uk); 2008. Accessed 1 August 2008.

37 Department for Children, Schools and Families. *The Children's Plan* (available at www.dcsf.gov.uk); 2007. Accessed 9 October 2008).

38 Office for Standards in Education (OFSTED). *Sex and Relationship Education.* London: HMSO, 2002.

39 DeBell D, Buttigieg M, Sherwin S, Lowe K. The school as a location for health promotion. In: DeBell D, ed. *Public Health Practice and the School Age Population.* London: Hodder Arnold, 2007.

40 Naidoo J, Wills J. *Health Promotion: Foundations for Practice,* 2nd edn. London: Baillere Tindall, 2000.

41 Lightfoot J, Bines W. *Keeping Children Healthy: The Role of School Nursing.* University of York: Social Policy Research Unit, 1997.

42 Department for Education and Skills (DfES). *National Healthy Schools Status: A Guide for Schools.* London: HMSO, 2005.

43 Mayall B. *Negotiating Health: Primary School Children at Home and School.* London: Cassell, 1994.

44 United Nations General Assembly resolution 44/25. *Convention on the Rights of the Child* (available at www.uncrc.info). Geneva: UN, 1989. Accessed 20 June 2008.

45 National Children's Bureau. *Children and Young People's Views on Health and Health Services: A Review of the Evidence.* London: NCB Publications, 2005.

46 Department for Children, Schools and Families. *The Children's Plan* (available at www.dcsf.gov.uk); 2007. Accessed 6 August 2008).

47 Department of Health. *Chief Nursing Officer's Review of the Nursing, Midwifery and Health Visiting Contribution to Vulnerable Children and Young People.* London: DH, 2004.

48 Department of Health. *You're Welcome Quality Criteria: Making Health Services Young People Friendly.* London: TSO, 2007.

49 *Education Act.* London: HMSO, 2002.

50 National Children's Bureau. *Developing a Whole School Approach to PSHE and Citizenship.* London: NCB Publications, 2003.

51 Nursing and Midwifery Council. *The Code: Standards of Conduct, Performance and Ethics for Nurses and Midwives* (available at www.nmc-uk.org). London: Nursing and Midwifery Council, 2008.

52 Social Science Research Unit. *NHS Teen LifeCheck Evaluation* (available at www.ioe.ac.uk/ssru). London: University of London, 2008. Accessed 30 July 2008.

53 Baptise L, Drennan V. Communication between school nurses and primary care teams. *British Journal of Community Nursing* 1999; **4**(1): 13-18.

54 *Children Act* (available at www.publications.parliament.uk); 2004. Accessed 30 April 2007.

55 National Governors' Association. *Extended Schools - A Guide for Governors 1.* Birmingham: National Remodelling Team, 2006.

56 Department for Education and Skills. *Extended Schools: Access to Opportunities and Services for All. A Prospectus.* Nottingham: DfES Publications, 2005.

57 Department of Health. *Extension of HPV Vaccination.* London: DH, 2008.

Chapter 7

What Is Occupational Health?

Greta Thornbory

Learning objectives

After reading this chapter you will be able to:

- Appreciate the role of occupational health (OH) in public health and how OH practice has evolved
- Appreciate the multidisciplinary approach of OH practice
- Identify the legal, financial and moral aspects and benefits of caring for worker's health
- Discuss the role of OH in workplace health promotion and the promotion of good health as good business

Introduction

This chapter will discuss OH and how it is related to public health. It will cover the objectives of an OH programme in the prevention of work-related ill health and the positive promotion of health, particularly in the United Kingdom (UK). It will explore the UK legal, as well as the financial and moral aspects of OH and the business world in which the OH professionals have to work as part of the multidisciplinary team, many of whom may not be health care professionals. It will highlight the importance of caring for the population of the workforce during its working life as a captive audience for health promotion.

OH is probably the least well known of the public health disciplines in health care. The name itself is often confused with occupational therapy, yet there is no comparison whatsoever with this branch of health care. OH is exactly what it says, the health of people in their occupations or work; another term which may serve to clarify its role is 'workplace health management' and there have been some moves to use this term [1] instead of OH in order to avoid confusion over the two disciplines.

Today, people in the UK may work from the age of 16 until they are well into old age. With changes taking place over retirement age through the Age Discrimination legislation [2] and, as the longevity of the population increases, people will be working for most of their lives and this may mean for more than 50 years. Even those who choose higher education and so defer 'starting work' undertake holiday, evening and weekend employment. People also spend one-third of their day working; so in a given 24-hour day we spend around 8 hours working and 8 hours sleeping; which leaves just 8 hours in which to do everything else including personal care, household chores, socialising and recreational activities. This means that work and the working environment are an important aspect of everybody's life and consequently 'work should do the worker no harm' a maxim enshrined by health and safety law in the UK. Research by Waddell and Burton [3] concludes that there is strong evidence that work is generally good for physical and mental health and well-being. OH is all about supporting this and helping employers and employees in 'workplace health management'. OH services are there to offer that help and support to the organisation and later in this chapter we will talk about the different ways in which OH services can offer that support.

The history of OH services

Because traditionally OH services were not a part of the UK NHS provision, it is often thought that it is a new branch of health care. However, there has been a long historical interest in the health and welfare of the workforce; there is mention of how work affects health in the Bible [4] and around that time, circa 3000 BC, there is evidence that in ancient Egypt when building the pyramids the slaves covered their mouths in order to prevent them inhaling the dust rising from the various building processes. In the eighteenth century, Dr Ramazinni, an Italian Professor of Medicine wrote his treatise on the diseases of workers, *De Morbis Artificum Diatriba* or Diseases of Tradesmen and Craftsmen [5], and is therefore regarded as the father of industrial medicine. In his work, he outlined the hazards to health of many substances, dusts, vapours and chemicals as well as other agents from some 52 occupations. Later, Charley in her interesting historical book explores the birth of industrial nursing and in particular the work of the nineteenth-century philanthropists who cared for their workers, not only from a health perspective but often also from a home and social aspect. It was here that OH nursing is thought to originate, from the work of Philippa Flowerday who worked in Norwich for Colman's Mustard and is attributed to be the first OH nurse, working in the mornings in the factory and in the afternoons with workers families – a sort of link between OH and health visiting! OH services were originally called 'industrial' medicine and nursing because of the advent of the industrial revolution in the eighteenth century when factory work was so very dangerous affecting the health and welfare of many people. This was not just adults either but also children; they were often given the most dangerous jobs that only small-sized people could do. In those days, and until the later part of the twentieth century, OH was not merely a preventative service but also acted as a casualty department which treated minor injuries and illnesses. More recently, treatment services have been discontinued in most UK OH services, particularly in light of the First Aid Regulations [6] and easier access to primary care and GPs through local health centres, although they continue on major building projects such as the recently completed Terminal 5 at Heathrow and the 2012 Olympic site.

In 1948, when the NHS started, it was recorded that 1944 people died per annum from accidents at work [7] – and that was only from those employers for whom statistics were kept – so that actual number was probably much higher. In 2006/2007, the figure had reduced to 241 people killed at work. Still too high, of course, but the improved health and safety legislation and better health of the population meant that the advice and care needed to prevent death had reduced significantly. However, there is a maxim that every business or employer requires 'maximum output for minimum outlay' from his workforce. Taking care of the health, safety and welfare of the workforce was, and still is, thought to be costly. However, today there is research [8–11] that shows that 'good health is good business' and, as will be seen later in the chapter, promoting a healthy workforce and taking an interest in health and well-being of employees can actually help to cut sickness absence rates, reduce accidents and prevent fatalities, therefore saving the employer money in the long run. Where the employer contributes towards a private health insurance plan they may also save money by improving the health of their workforce, and help to avoid costly early retirement on the grounds of ill health. Savings to the pension fund are a benefit to all of those who contribute.

Hence, industrial health was born out of an industrial age. In the latter half of the twentieth century there has been a decrease in manufacturing, a growth in the service industries and the globalisation of enterprises in the business arena; this together with the advent of computers and other technologies, the name was changed from 'industrial' to 'occupational' health and in 1950 the Joint ILO (International Labour Organization)/WHO (World Health Organization) issued the first definition of OH which was updated in 1995 to these three objectives:

(1) The maintenance and promotion of workers' health and working capacity
(2) The improvement of working environment and work to become conducive to health and safety
(3) The development of work organisation and working cultures in a direction which supports health and safety at work and in doing so promotes a positive social climate and smooth operation and may enhance the productivity of the undertaking

Twelfth Session of the Joint ILO/WHO Committee on Occupational Health 1995

In 2002, the WHO Regional Office for Europe [12] produced guidance for OH professionals and outlined the 11 key functions of an OH service:

Functions of OH services:

(1) Identification and assessment of the health risk in the workplace
(2) Surveillance of work environment factors and work practices that affect workers' health, including sanitary installations, canteens and housing, when such facilities are provided by the employer
(3) Participation in the development of programmes for the improvement of working practices, as well as testing and evaluating health aspects of new equipment
(4) Advice on planning and organisation of work, design of workplaces, choice and maintenance of machinery, equipment and substances used at work
(5) Advice on OH, safety and hygiene, and on ergonomics and individual and collective protective equipment
(6) Surveillance of workers' health in relation to work
(7) Promoting the adaptation of work to the worker
(8) Collaboration in providing information, training and education in the fields of OH, hygiene and ergonomics
(9) Contribution to measures of vocational rehabilitation
(10) Organisation of first-aid and emergency treatment
(11) Participation in the analysis of occupational accidents and occupational diseases

It should be remembered that these key functions related to OH throughout the European Union (EU) and that many countries in the EU have vastly different health care services and are at different stages of development following the political changes over the last 20 years. There is also a diverse team of OH professionals who undertake this work and it is not just doctors and nurses involved in delivering these 11 functions.

Activity 7.1

Make a list of all the different disciplines you consider are involved with the health and well-being of people in the workplace. Consider how many of them are health care professionals? Then decide what you believe is a health care professional. See if you can find a definition. There is one on the Health Protection Agency website.

Delivering OH services

In most large organisations, i.e. those employing more than 250 employees, there is a department that is responsible for the human resources or personnel that the company employs; however, in many small- or medium-sized enterprises (SMEs) the employer accepts responsibility and undertakes this work himself. The EU has started to standardise the concept of SMEs to avoid confusion. Its current definition categorises companies with fewer than 50 employees as 'small', and those with fewer than 250 as 'medium' [13].

In 2006, there were 4.5m businesses in the UK of which only 0.1% employed more than 250 people [14]. This means that there are few 'in-house' OH services and a great need for SMEs to have access to some form of OH advice and support to care for the health of people at work. So, whilst the employer is always responsible for the OH and safety of his staff, in many organisations OH really begins with the person responsible for the 'human' resources or 'personnel' within the organisation. Where there is a human resources department (HR) then they are usually responsible for employing the OH service and personnel and in turn the OH service personnel are answerable to HR. This is often controversial as there are schools of thought amongst OH professionals that OH services should be totally independent and answerable directly to the employer or the Board of Directors, depending on the status and structure of the organisation. However, the recent report on the review of the health of Britain's working population by Dame Carol Black [15] says that *'developing an integrated approach to working-age health requires occupational health to be brought into mainstream health care provision'* and a number of pilot studies along these lines are to be set up in the UK during the next few years and it is worth keeping an eye out in the professional journals for updates on this initiative. At the time of writing there are discussions taking place on developing a Council of Occupational Health bringing together the various disciplines involved in OH.

So, who exactly is part of the OH team and who is an OH professional? Box 7.1 shows most of the OH team but it is not exclusive.

Box 7.1   The occupational health team

Occupational health physician
Occupational health nurse
Occupational health technician
Occupational hygienist
Occupational psychologist
Counsellors
Ergonomists
Health and safety adviser or manager
Case managers
Fire safety specialist
Manual handling adviser
Physiotherapist
Administrative or clerical support

All these people contribute to the health, safety and well-being of people at work and may be employed by the company on a permanent, sessional or advisory capacity. There is no law that says any of them should be employed but it is interesting to note that at a recent employment tribunal, when Dundee City Council were found in breach of the Management of Health and Safety Regulations, the personnel manager admitted that he did not understand the meaning of OH and the tribunal itself struggled to define it during the course of the hearing [16]. It would probably have been better if they had asked for an OH expert from one of the OH bodies (see appendix) to give an explanation and to demonstrate the business case. This serves to demonstrate that not having access to OH advice can result in legal action being taken. Whilst the various regulations in the area of health and safety do not require organisations to employ specifically OH professionals, they do require that certain services, such as risk assessment and health surveillance, are provided by competent persons, and it is the employers' duty to ensure that the people that they employ are competent.

The OH team is made up of both OH health care professionals and others who are not regarded as health care professionals. A health care professional is distinguished by the fact that their profession is regulated by statute and is either a member of the Health Professions Council (HPC; www.hpc-uk.org), the Nursing and Midwifery Council (NMC) or the General Medical Council (GMC). All these health care professions have a code of profession practice and must respect patient/client confidentiality. This is the main difference between the OH health care professional and the other OH professionals and members of the OH team. Which members of the OH team are employed, and whether on a permanent or advisory basis, will depend on the specific company, its type, size and the work that it does. There is no set model for an OH team. There is a great deal of overlap between the different members of the team and there are times when this may cause problems. Smedley et al. [17] say that provided role definitions are clear and overlaps and gaps are managed sensitively any combination can be successful. It is useful to describe the different roles.

OH physicians

OH physicians are qualified doctors and occupational medicine (OM) is a recognised branch of clinical medicine. The principal role of OM is the provision of health advice to organisations and individuals. There are several levels of specialist training in OM a qualified doctor can undertake, depending on what aspect of OH he/she wishes to be involved. A general practitioner may wish to offer specialist services to local companies as part of his GP work; to do this, he should achieve the basic level of qualification which is the Diploma in Occupational Medicine. This will enable him to understand the main issues affecting health and work and to appreciate the difference between caring for a healthy population of a workforce and the clinical role of the GP for individual patients. To become an associate member of the Faculty of Occupational Medicine the doctor will need to study an agreed training programme and this is aimed at doctors interested in pursuing a full-time career in OM and they must demonstrate a core knowledge in OM theory and practice. To obtain consultant status in OM or Membership of the Faculty of Occupational Medicine they must achieve the Higher Specialist Training by undertaking accredited courses and complete a dissertation which must be accepted (www.som.org.uk).

OH nurses

OH nurses are nurses who have studied a specific course and who work at a specialist level in public health nursing. They must meet the standards for entry to be part of the specialist community public health nurse (SCPHN) register. A nurse must be on the nursing part of the NMC Register to be eligible for entry to the SCPHN part (see Chapter 2). The NMC (www.nmc-uk.org) say that all nurses have a role to play in promoting the public's health, but that only a proportion of them will work at a level where they can promote change by working in partnership with a wide range of agencies, making decisions that influence whole populations. Employers are under no legal obligation to employ qualified OH nurses, but if nurses take on work they are not qualified to do they would be in breach of their professional code; the NMC code [18] says that you must have *the knowledge and skills for safe and effective practice when working without direct supervision* and that you must *recognise and work within the limits of your competence*. Failure to do so could result in suspension of your registration and therefore licence to practice. Further, more in-depth, explanations of OH nursing will be given in Chapter 8.

OH technicians

OH technicians are much like health care assistants. They are trained to carry out specific basic OH tasks – often repetitive or straightforward things such as audiometry or lung function testing – and may not even have a health background. They are expected to work within closely defined protocols and procedures, but are not expected to make clinical judgements and they are usually answerable to a qualified OH nurse or physician. There are specific courses for OH technicians – see appendix.

Occupational hygienist

Occupational hygiene is about recognising, evaluating and controlling health hazards arising from work. Occupational hygienists have an in-depth knowledge of how chemical, physical and biological agents may affect the health of the workforce, and in turn the health of the business. They advise on controlling health risks by assessing and resolving practical problems in all types of workplaces. A qualified occupational hygienist has undertaken a suitable higher education course recognised for entry to the British Occupational Hygiene Society (BOHS). Only very large organisations or those with specific hazards and risk would employ an occupational hygienist full time, so many consultancies exist for employers to call on their expertise as and when needed (see appendix for more details).

Ergonomists

Ergonomics is the application of scientific information concerning humans to the design of objects, systems and environment for human use [19]. Ergonomists ensure that equipment, facilities and systems are designed and organised to the highest standards of comfort, efficiency, health and safety for the people using them. By scientifically studying the relationship between people, environments and equipment, ergonomists can use their findings to improve human interaction with processes/systems. Areas of work include product/equipment design, production systems, information and advanced technology, and transport design. They may work in consultancy, research, development or teaching and may also be called human factors specialists. Ergonomics comes into everything which involves people. Work systems, sports and leisure, health and safety should all embody ergonomics principles if well designed. There are different levels of qualification from student, graduate through to fellow and honorary fellow. Again, only large organisations with specific hazards and risk would usually employ an occupational hygienist full time, so consultancies exist for employers to call on their expertise when needed (see appendix for more details).

Occupational psychologists

Occupational psychologists are specialist psychologists who apply psychological knowledge, theory and practice to the world of work. They determine how work conditions and tasks can affect people by developing or constraining them and influencing their well-being, and on how individuals and their characteristics determine what work is done, and how. They may work in a consultancy role, or maybe employed within a large organisation working with management, training officers etc. and work both with teams and individual staff.

Counsellors

Counselling is one of the talking therapies and at the moment is not a health care profession although there are moves to regulate the discipline when it will become one of the professions regulated by the HPC. The British Association for Counselling and Psychotherapy (BACP) offers an accreditation scheme (MBACP) for counsellors. It requires prospective counsellors to accrue at least 450 hours in both theoretical and practical training. Counsellors actually help people to explore feelings about their lives so that they can reflect about what is happening to them and consider alternative ways of doing things. It is a confidential service as counsellors listen attentively to their clients and offer them the time, empathy and respect they need to express their own feelings in a safe environment. Counselling is an important aspect of OH as one of the biggest causes of sickness absence from work is stress-related illness, particularly mental ill health. Businesses are encouraged by the Health and Safety Executive to employ the services of 'employee assistance programmes' (EAPs) which offers confidential services to employees.

Health and safety

Employers must designate someone in their organisation to be responsible for the health and safety arrangements [20]. The type of organisation, the hazards and the risks to health and safety will usually determine the quality of the post holder. The person may be called an adviser, officer, manager etc. and there is no control over the qualifications or experience this person will need to have; and when they do have them, health and safety qualifications do not make the person a health care professional.

Regulation 7 of the Management of health and safety at work Regulation [20] states 'Every employer shall, ... appoint one or more competent persons to assist him in undertaking the measures he needs to take to comply... with the relevant statutory provisions' and 'a person shall be regarded as competent... where he has sufficient training and experience or knowledge and other qualities to properly assist in the undertaking'. The guidance goes on to say that competence in this case does not necessarily mean possession of qualifications but more complicated organisations will require the 'competent' person to have a higher level of knowledge and experience or they may have particular technical knowledge and experience of a specific process or substance. The lack of control over this role has sometimes meant that qualified OH nurses are answerable to less qualified health and safety personnel, or they are answerable to qualified health and safety people who lack understanding of OH and the role of the OH nurse; this has on occasions led to conflict.

Today, a number of organisations offer training courses at various levels, from certificate through to masters degree, but the recognised leading body on health and safety is the Institute of Occupational Safety and Health (IOSH) where those people who have undertaken suitable training and have obtained the necessary qualifications can register to become members etc. and continuing professional development must be demonstrated in order to maintain membership - see appendix.

Case managers

According to the Case Management Society (www.cmsuk.org), the role of a case manager is to collaborate with clients by assessing, facilitating, planning and advocating for health and social needs on an individual basis. They go on to define case management as:

A collaborative process which assesses, plans, implements, co-ordinates, monitors and evaluates the options and services required to meet an individuals health, care, educational and employment needs, using communication and available resources to promote quality cost effective outcomes.

Of course, much of the work of an OH nurse could be said to be that of case management, but case managers may also be non-health care professionals, although they do need appropriate qualifications and experience and the society lays down standards and has an approved code of ethics [21]. The Case Management Society say that case management originated in the United States. In the past, providers of services have been mainly community nurses and social workers who coordinated their services through the public health sector. More recently, insurance companies have employed nurses and social workers to assist with the coordination of care for people who have suffered complex injuries requiring multidisciplinary intervention. EEF [22] suggest that a case management approach to sickness absence is the way forward and that line managers are best placed to fill such a role.

Fire safety specialist

This role is often combined with that of Safety Officer except where there is a specific type of fire risk.

Manual handling adviser

This role is found most frequently in the NHS where patient handling is a major area of concern both for the health and safety of employees and patients alike.

Physiotherapist

Chartered physiotherapists are often employed by large companies on a sessional basis in order to get employees with work and non-work, often sports, injuries back to work quickly. Musculoskeletal disorders (MSDs) are the most common cause of sickness absence and the Chief Executive of the Chartered Institute of Physiotherapists says that 'Physiotherapists are ideally placed to tackle workplace ill health and help keep people in work. By intervening early, and playing a key role in the treatment and prevention of health conditions that affect ability to work, physiotherapists can improve patient health and well-being and reduce benefit dependency'.

Administrative or clerical support

A vital role is that of the OH department's clerical support staff. However, as they are not health care professionals they should sign a confidentiality declaration.

From this explanation of the 'OH Team', it is clear that OH help and advice can be delivered by a wide and diverse range of people.

Good health is good business: the legal aspects

Or so it is said and has been shown by various pieces of research quoted earlier in the chapter. However, employers want maximum output for minimum outlay and in the UK they expect the NHS to take care of their employee's health. There is a great deal of case law that shows that employers have not always taken care of employees' health and in fact one of the gold standard cases in 1968 [23] confirms that the courts felt that the company ought to have known and dealt with the risk to the health of the employees [24]. There have been numerous subsequent cases illustrating that employers still do not always take care of their employee's health, safety and welfare. Back in 1968, there was a great deal of piecemeal legislation dating back over a hundred years and in 1974, following the Robens Report, the most significant piece of health and safety legislation became law – The Health and Safety at Work etc. Act 1974.

The Health and Safety at Work etc. Act

The Health and Safety at Work etc. Act (HASAWA) is an enabling act; in other words, it acts as an umbrella so that other secondary legislations or regulations can be made under this 'Act of Parliament'. The most significant aspect of the Act is that it covers all employees (except domestic servants) for the first time ever and in Section 2, it places responsibility for the health, safety and welfare of employees, as far as is reasonably practicable, squarely on the shoulders of the employer. It also requires employers to provide safe systems of working, as well as adequate training and supervision [25]. The phrase 'as far as reasonably practicable' has been defined in law [26]. Anyone in breach of the Act is subject to punishment through criminal prosecution and many prosecutions have taken place over the intervening years; examples of these can be seen by visiting the Health and Safety Executive website (www.hse.gov.uk/enforce/index.htm; last accessed 29 July 2008). Employers often believe that they have insurance that will cover such prosecutions, which is not the case, and we will deal with this in more depth later in the chapter under financial aspects. They may also require help and advice with regard to ensuring the health, safety and welfare at work of his employees and this is where the OH team come in. Note that the OH team offer help and advice, they do not take over responsibility; that remains firmly with the employer who may choose not to take the OH help and advice offered.

Risk assessment

Since 1974, there have been many regulations made under the Act but probably one of the most significant is the Management of Health and Safety at Work Regulations 1999 (MHSW) originally made in 1992 as part of what was known as the 'six pack' or 6 pieces of health and safety legislations passed to bring UK legislation into line with a European health and safety directive. This has, at times, mistakenly been called European legislation. The MHSW requires all employers to undertake a 'risk assessment' of the undertaking as the risks to health and safety vary according to the type and place of work; for ease of identification, this is often known as the four Ps:

- **P**remises
- **P**lant (or equipment)
- **P**rocesses
- **P**eople

The risk assessment requires employers to determine the hazards and therefore the risks to the safety and health of the employees; the Health and Safety Executive give five stages to the risk assessment:

(1) Identify the hazard(s) to health and safety
(2) Quantify the risk – who might be hurt and how
(3) Put in place measures to eliminate, reduce or control the risks to health and safety
(4) Record findings and details of control measures
(5) Review periodically, such as when new equipment is installed or when working practices change – but at least once a year

Various members of the OH team may be needed to offer help and advice with regard to the risk assessment and putting in place suitable control measures. A simple example of a risk assessment in an office environment is given here, as almost every workplace will have some type of office (see Figure 7.1).

Activity 7.2

Undertake a risk assessment: See if you can spot the hazards and estimate the risks to health and safety in Figure 7.1. Then compare your findings with the text below.

(1) Identify the hazards: Offices are regarded as fairly safe places to work and therefore low risk. However, there are a few areas where problems may occur. Considering the four Ps we need to look at the office itself then at the plant or equipment in the room and the work that is undertaken using that equipment. The increased use of computers over the past 30 years has brought about concerns with eyes and eyesight, and concentrated time spent in front of a computer screen (known as 'display screen equipment' or DSE) has proved to cause various MSDs. In this picture, the office worker is using a laptop computer and, despite the relaxed looking position, the man is at risk of developing upper limb MSDs. Also in the

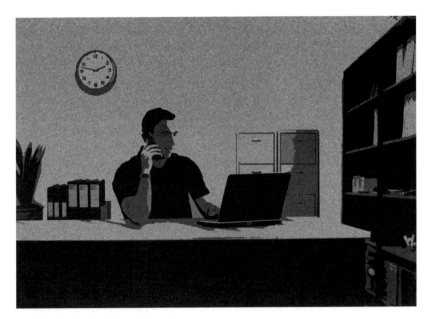

Figure 7.1

picture there are filing cabinets, these can be loaded unevenly and may topple open when draws are open, or people may trip over drawers left open. Finally, the bookcase on the right has some high shelves, reaching for high storage can be hazardous and also cause MSDs.

(2) Quantify the risk, who might be hurt and why: Obviously, the man himself is at risk of MSDs and anyone who visits his office could be hurt by tripping over open drawers of the filing cabinet.

(3) Put in place measures to eliminate, reduce or control the risks to health and safety: The DSE regulations and the HSE guidance on the regulations [27] require that the man in the picture needs to be made aware of the risks to his health. He needs to be shown or receive training on how to adjust his workstation to his individual needs in order to prevent MSDs. Where this is not possible the employer must provide suitable adjustments to provide an ergonomically sound work station. His work processes should be such that he is able to spend time on other work away from the DSE or at least have a very short break every 50 minutes.

According to the Regulations, he should be able to request an eye test by a competent person and for the employer to pay for suitable corrective lenses if ordinary corrective lenses are not sufficient.

Under health and safety legislation, an employer must also provide suitable training and supervision for all health and safety hazards and that would include advice on using filing cabinets and storage.

(4) Record these findings and the details of control measures.

(5) Review periodically – such as when new equipment is installed or when working practices change – but at least once a year.

> ## Activity 7.3
>
> Now undertake a risk assessment at your place of work, probably your own office, workstation or clinic area would be a good place to start. Then compare this with the company risk assessments

Employment law

Under the Employment Rights Act 1996, employees have the right not to be dismissed unfairly from their jobs. In order for employers to act fairly and reasonably with their employees they will need the help and advice of an OH health care professional to give advice particularly when there is a question of ill health or capability [24].

Employers believe that they should employ people that are 'fit' to do the work but what exactly does 'fit' mean? Like health it is a concept and much has been written about exactly who or what defines health [28], but employers expect someone to say 'this person is fit to work' or not. However, much will depend on the type of job, where and how the work is done and what it involves. Only when the 'risk assessment' for that job has been undertaken, can it be decided what health and fitness criteria are needed to assess an individual's fitness or otherwise for such work. So when an employee is returning from long-term sick leave or has taken frequent short spells of sickness absence the work that that person is doing will need to be assessed along with their mental and physical ability or otherwise to do the work. Care must be taken by the employer because of the Disability Discrimination Act (DDA).

DDA 1995

This Act makes it an offence to discriminate against somebody because they are disabled. The word 'disabled' often conjures up images of a person in a wheelchair but the meaning of disability under the Act is much broader than that (see Box 7.2).

Employers must make reasonable adjustments for employees, either existing or prospective, if it is thought that it is likely they will come under the DDA. There are several significant points here:

(1) OH professionals can only make recommendations to employers as to whether they consider someone would be likely to come under the DDA; they are not in a position to state categorically as that is the prerogative of the courts.
(2) The law requires employers to make 'reasonable' adjustments and, as Lewis [24] says, the word is subject to constant legal argument. Reasonable may be considered in the terms of the cost to the employer and the impact it may have on the workplace and other employees, as well as the impact on the process of work that is undertaken.

Box 7.2 Disability Discrimination Act definitions

The statutory definition of disability discrimination is when:

A person directly discriminates against a disabled person, if, on the grounds of the disabled person's disability, he treats the disabled person less favourably than he treats or would treat a person not having that particular disability whose relevant circumstances, including his abilities are the same as, or not materially different from, those of the disabled person.

A person has a disability according to the DDA if:

He has a physical or mental impairment which has a substantial and long-term adverse effect on his ability to carry out normal day-to-day activities.

---

(3) Most significantly adjustments can be quite simple, such as adjusting work hours or seeking help and advice from specific bodies, such as Access to Work or Royal National Institute of Blind People – see appendix for further information. They do not have to involve 'unreasonable' amounts of outlay.

(4) According to the DDA (see Box 7.2) a person will be considered to have a disability if it interferes with his or her ability to carry out normal day-to-day activities. Activities of daily living are the things we normally do day to day and they include such things as eating, washing, dressing, grooming, working, homemaking and leisure. OH nurses may like to consider the Roper, Tierney and Logan model of 'Activities for Daily Living' [29] to help put this into some sort of perspective. Here Roper et al. outline the factors that influence the activities of daily living as:

- Physical
- Psychological
- Sociocultural
- Environmental
- Politicoeconomic

And this fits well with the biopsychosocial model considered today which will be discussed in the next chapter.

The Data Protection Act 1998

In seeking to employ someone or to find out if an employee, or prospective employee, is fit to do the work it is necessary to gather information about that person, in other words, to gather 'personal data' which will need to be processed, used and stored. The Data Protection Act (DPA) says that there are two different types of personal data – the straightforward personal data of name and address etc. and then sensitive personal data which include such things as ethnic origin, gender, religious beliefs and information about a person's mental or physical health. Sensitive data can only be held with the consent of the person to whom the data relates. It is this 'sensitive' data to which OH records and medical information relates.

The DPA is comprehensive and has eight main principles (www.ico.gov.uk) to make sure that personal data are:

- Fairly and lawfully processed
- Processed for limited purposes
- Adequate, relevant and not excessive
- Accurate and up to date
- Not kept for longer than is necessary
- Processed in line with your rights
- Secure
- Not transferred to other countries without adequate protection

This is very significant in OH practice especially as any personal data that is gathered must be 'adequate, relevant and not excessive'. That means that health questions should only be asked that have a significant bearing on the employment of that individual. This will be discussed in more depth in the next chapter when considering pre-employment health assessment, but questions about family history, for example, generally have no place in OH practice.

Personal data should be 'not kept for longer than necessary' and there are guidelines for keeping certain health and medical records in other legislation, such as the Control of Substances Hazardous to Health Regulations 2002 which requires health surveillance records to be kept for 40 years.

The Information Commissioner has produced a valuable 'Employment Practices Code' [30] in four parts:

(1) Recruitment and selection
(2) Employment records
(3) Monitoring at work
(4) Workers' health

This code can be downloaded free from the Information Commissioners website and gives guidance on the handling of sensitive data.

Other legislation which is relevant to the work of the OH nurse will be discussed later in the chapter on OH nursing.

Good health is good business: the financial aspects

A business's most valuable asset is . . . the dedicated staff that devotes themselves to delivering the work of the organisation. Healthy and fit staff are essential to ensuring a company remains efficient and profitable.

(Professor Dame Carol Black [31])

So it is well recognised that the health and welfare of the individual employees plays a great part in the success or otherwise of the company and therefore there are financial reasons for ensuring that fitness. Employers are required by law to pay the Employers Liability Compulsory Insurance (ELCI) and, as mentioned before, employers often quote that they have this insurance and paid their premium so are covered for should anything happen to them which will cost. The premium is to cover injuries and ill heath experienced by employees whilst at work. However, it does not cover all the costs. For every £1 of insured costs of an accident or ill health there will be another £10 of uninsured costs (www.hse.gov.uk/costs). The ELCI will not cover:

- Sick pay to employees
- Damage or loss of product or raw materials
- Repairs to machinery or equipment
- Overtime, temporary or agency workers needed to cover the work of sick or injured employees
- Delays in production
- Time taken for investigation by health and safety, HR, line managers
- Fines, court costs and any excess on claims
- Loss of further business and reputation

The HSE say that ELCI only pays out the tip of the iceberg. So costs of ill health and accidents may be considerable. Pickvance [8] says that the evidence that employers can reduce or control insurance costs by improving health and safety is debatable. The exception is where there are specific problems when fear of litigation costs and therefore increased insurance premiums, has encouraged employers to improve preventative measures. Research [32] found that workers' compensation arrangements in other countries positively motivated health and safety arrangements and rehabilitation. The research concluded that there is evidence that a reform of the UK insurance process would provide significant motivation for employers to improve health, safety and rehabilitation. Wright [9] said that since 2002 employers have been experiencing the true cost of liability insurance and that this is the result of poor investment in the market with the knock-on effect that insurers raise their premiums. Add this to the higher compensation costs and health care costs the result is that employers have to pay even higher premiums. Insurers have now moved to 'risk-based' pricing of insurance and employers now have to take the issue of OH and health and safety in hand to keep premiums as low as possible.

Another study [10] examined a number of case studies that provide evidence of the business benefits of OH and safety interventions (Table 7.1). Every one of those reasons listed in Table 7.1 has a financial implication. It must be remembered that the average recruitment cost of filling an employee vacancy is over £4000 and in some instances this increases to nearly £8000 [33].

Table 7.1 Examples of business benefits arising from health and safety interventions.

Direct benefits	Indirect benefits
Reduced insurance premiums	Reduced absenteeism
Reduced litigation costs	Reduced staff turnover
Reduced sick pay costs	Improved corporate image
Improved production/productivity rates	Improved chance of winning contracts
Lower accident costs/production delays	Improved job satisfaction/morale
Reduced product and material damage	

There is an extremely high cost from unplanned sickness absence and one of the biggest roles of an OH service is its involvement with advising and supporting the employer in managing absence. Indeed OH services have been quoted by both the Confederation of British Industry (CBI) and the Chartered Institute of Personnel and Development (CIPD) as the most effective way of dealing with sickness absence through early referral. The most recent report from CIPD [34] quotes the use of OH services as most highly rated for both short-term and long-term absence.

Health promotion

If good health is good business and work is good for health then the employee is a captive audience for health promotion. Professor Dame Carol Black recently published her review of the health of Britain's working-age population [15] in which she said that improving the health of the working-age population was critically important to secure higher economic growth and increased social justice. Among her objectives were the prevention of illness and the promotion of health and well-being together with early intervention for those who develop a health condition. She goes on to highlight that legislation has played a part in improving health and safety at work and that a new approach to health and well-being is needed; she makes suggestions about the way forward and that OH should be brought under the main stream health care provision. She also proposes a new 'fit for work' service, with several different models tested and evaluated over the next few years. This is all in the pipeline, but what is happening out there now?

Health promotion is about promoting health living and if we revisit the day-to-day activities of living of eating, washing, dressing, grooming, working, homemaking and leisure and, bearing in mind we spend one-third of our life at work, then many of these aspects of our daily life occur at, or through, work. Kreis and Bödeker [35] say that workplace health promotion programmes actually prove to be more effective than community programmes. They also suggest that such programmes lead to a reduction in absenteeism and provide a return of investment. The WHO in their Declaration on Workers Health [36] in 2006 state that there is growing recognition about the linkages between working conditions, health and productivity and that primary prevention of disease is cost-effective; they go on to say that to achieve this requires a holistic approach combining OH with disease prevention, health promotion and tackling the social determinants of health.

> ### Activity 7.4
>
> Consider what you can do to help promote a healthy workforce bearing in mind your time and financial constraints then compare your answers with the suggestions below.

In light of all the above it is worth considering what has been achieved already and the contribution that can be made by organisations for their employees, particularly on the key topics identified in Chapter 2.

Smoking

Already with recent legislation smoking has been banned in all enclosed public places since July 2007. To assist with this a number of initiatives to support employers and employees alike have been available and the report [37] from the government on the first 12 months is encouraging and positive. The initiative seems to be working.

Healthy eating

The government statistics (www.foresight.gov.uk) on obesity show that there is wide spread obesity and this needs to be tackled. The government project 'Foresight' aims to 'to produce a long-term vision of how they can deliver a sustainable response to obesity in the UK over the next 40 years'. This is at a national level, but at a local employment level much can be done at work to improve the diets of working people by:

- Making sure employees take regular breaks especially away from their work stations
- Providing pleasant areas in which to take breaks to eat and drink
- Ensuring there is an adequate supply of fresh drinking water (this is a legal requirement under the workplace) Health, Safety and Welfare Regulations 1992
- Offering healthy choices of food. Tea trolleys and canteens should be offering fresh fruit and vegetables and cutting down on salt and fried or fatty food

- Automatic vending machines should be regularly stocked with healthier alternatives to chocolate bars and fizzy drinks
- Departments should allocate the tea and coffee money to fresh fruit rather than packets of biscuits

Physical activity

More and more work these days is of a sedentary nature and even in manufacturing much is done by robots. For people in those sedentary jobs there is a need to get some exercise to improve and maintain a healthy cardiovascular system, prevent obesity and MSDs. MSDs are one of the two top reasons for long-term sickness absence, the other being stress-related illness. It is said that exercise is also good for relieving stress, the other main reason for sickness absence.

OH services can do a lot to advice employers on suitable ways of supporting employees in increasing people's activity. Playtex (or DB Apparel) is a case study example of a company taking onboard advise to improve employee morale. They started the annual power walking event 'Playtex Moon Walk' to raise funds for a breast cancer charity. In doing so they generated energy and motivation among their staff and have subsequently built on that. Originally, 49% of staff were not exercising at all and now 68% are engaged in exercise [38].

Employers can help employees with their physical fitness in many ways. Here are a few suggestions:

- Arranging for cheap rate membership to local sports clubs and gyms, or even provide in-house facilities if possible
- Make available information on local sports activities, clubs etc. and the benefits of physical activity
- Encourage inter-workplace or departmental teams for sports activities both inside and outside working hours
- Encourage employees to walk or cycle to work. To promote healthier journeys to work and reduce environmental pollution, the 1999 Finance Act introduced an annual tax exemption, which allows employers to loan cycles and cyclists' safety equipment to employees as a tax-free benefit (www.dft.gov.uk). The exemption was one of a series of measures introduced under the government's 'Green Transport Plan'. So there are several companies that offer to work with employers in supplying bicycles under this scheme, such as www.cyclescheme.co.uk
- Employees are allowed by law to take regular breaks away from their workstation. The Working Time Regulations require that employers give rest breaks of not less than 20 minutes if working longer than 6 hours; this length is increased to 30 minutes after 4½ hours for young people
- Make sure people take their annual leave entitlement

Alcohol and drug misuse

It seems strange to put drugs and alcohol together as one is a legal substance and other is illegal. Today, there are government-recommended limits for alcohol consumption and it has to be remembered that what a person does in their own time is not the province of the employer. It becomes his province when abuse of these substances impact on the working environment and put people at risk to their health and safety, the Information Commissioner gives more details on this topic especially from the ethics and data protection viewpoint of testing for drugs and alcohol in the workplace (www.ico.gov.uk). From a health promotion perspective it is advisable for employers to have policies and procedures in place to deal with drug and alcohol misuse. The role of the OH nurse in drugs and alcohol misuse will be covered in more detail in the next chapter.

Mental well-being

According to national surveys, the main causes of absence from work are back pain, MSDs and stress [34, 39]. Work-related stress accounts for over one-third of all new incidences of ill health and that each case of stress-related ill health leads to an average of 30.9 working days lost (www.hse.gov.uk/stress). This means that over 12.8 million working days are lost per annum due to stress, depression and anxiety. There are also other mental health conditions with which employees may suffer including schizophrenia, bi-polar disorders (manic depression) psychosis, obsessive compulsive disorders and eating disorders. It goes to show that maintaining mental well-being is an important aspect of employment and it is worth employers investing in suitable health promotion activities. Mindful Employer (www.mindfulemployer.net), an organisation led by employers, for employers and set up by the NHS says that if given the right support people with mental health conditions are able to stay at work.

The HSE define stress as *'The adverse reaction people have to excessive pressure or other types of demand placed on them'*. According to ACAS, stress is often a symptom of poor employment relations and can seriously affect productivity. To help prevent work-related stress the HSE have published a set of evidence-based standards recommended for employers to follow. These standards are about helping employers to prevent mental ill health and require commitment of at all levels or the organisation. The research showed that there are six key areas of work design which, if not properly managed, may lead to ill health, reduced productivity and increased sickness absence. In each area a risk assessment should be carried out to cover these points:

- **Demands**: What are the demands of the job? Can the employees cope?
- **Control**: To what degree do employees have control over their work? Does management consult with employees so that they can have a say in how they should go about their work?

- **Support**: What level of management and colleague support is provided? Are employees provided with information and support? Are policies and procedures easily accessible? Are they given regular and constructive feedback?
- **Relationships**: What is the quality of work relationships? Has the organisation addressed and eliminated workplace intimidation and bullying?
- **Role**: Is the employee aware of his/her role within the organisation and how it is managed?
- **Change**: How is change managed? Is there sufficient communication with employees? Do they have any involvement with change?

What can an employer do?

- The HSE website recommends a risk assessment and offers downloadable guidance for doing this.
- Put in place suitable policies and procedures relevant to stress and mental health.
- Make sure managers are trained to manage people, not just the process. Then make sure they have adequate information and training about stress and other mental health issues and how to deal with them.
- OH professionals can help with raising awareness and understanding of mental health issues in the workplace amongst the workforce.
- Employers need to make sure employees have access to an Employee Assistance Programme (EAP). EAP's services are usually free to the employee. These are often via contracts with an independent EAP company. This is also a confidential service so employers do not know who is using their employee assistance programmes, unless there are extenuating circumstances and the proper release forms have been signed.

Summary

This chapter has attempted to explain what OH is and what it is not. Health and safety at work is the employers' responsibility and also everybody's business; therefore, good health means good business. The chapter has also discussed the various disciplines that go to make up the team of people who contribute to workplace health and who advise employers on all aspects of OH matters.

Much of workplace health is governed by, or impinged on by statutory requirements and mandatory guidance, so the legislation and legal aspects have been explored in the most significant legislation. For more in-depth details on relevant law and in particular, case law, it is best to look at a textbook on that subject [24]. There are substantial financial benefits to employers who show consideration for the health of their employees. These are evident from the research that has shown how employment and the place of work can contribute to health promotion in the workforce and therefore the health of the nation.

References

1 Whitaker S, Baranski B. *The Role of the Occupational Health Nurse in Workplace Health Management.* Geneva: WHO, 2001.

2 The Employment Equality (Age) Regulations 2006, SI No 1031.

3 Waddell G, Burton AK. *Is Work Good for Your Health and Wellbeing?* London: TSO, 2006.

4 Ecclesiasticus 38 v25-35.

5 Charley I. *The Birth of Industrial Nursing: Its History and Development in Great Britain.* London: Balliere, Tindall and Cox, 1954.

6 Health and Safety (First Aid) Regulations 1981 SI No. 917.

7 Gifford P. From phenol poisoning to stress: 60 years of health and safety. *Health Care Risk Report* 2008; **14**(8): 18-19.

8 Pickvance S. Arguing the business case for occupational health. *Occupational Health Review* 2003; **May/June**(103): 31-5.

9 Wright M. *The Business Case in Well-Being at Work.* London: IOD, 2006.

10 Shearn P. Case Examples: Business Benefits Arising from Health and Safety Interventions (HSL/2003/13), 2003.

11 Hu Tec Associates Ltd. *The Cost and Benefits of Active Case Management and Rehabilitation for Musculoskeletal Disorders* (available at www.hse.gov.uk/research.rrhtm/rr493.htm); 2006.

12 Lie A, Baranski B, Husman K, Westerholm P. *Good Practice in Occupational Health Services: A Contribution to Workplace Health.* Copenhagen: WHO Regional Office, 2002.

13 European Commission (2003-05-06), *Recommendation 2003/361/EC: SME Definition* (available at http://europa.eu.int/comm/enterprise/enterprise_policy/sme_definition/index_en.htm). Accessed on 15 July 2008.

14 Department for Business, Enterprise and Regulatory Reform. *National Statistics* (available at http://stats.berr.gov.uk/ed/sme/smestats2006-ukspr.pdf).

15 Black C. *Working for a Healthier Tomorrow: A Review of the Health of Britain's Working Age Population* (available at www.workingforhealth.gov.uk); 2008.

16 Tribunal dismisses appeal against 'disproportionate' HSE action. *Occupational Health Review* 2006; **Nov/Dec**(124).

17 Smedley J, Dick F, Sadhra S. *Oxford Handbook of Occupational Health.* Oxford: Oxford University Press, 2007.

18 Nursing and Midwifery Council. *The Code: Standards of Conduct, Performance and Ethics for Nurses and Midwives.* London: NMC, 2008.

19 Ergonomics Society (available at www.ergonomics.org.uk). Accessed 24 July 2008.

20 HSE. *Management of Health and Safety at Work.* Approved Code of Practice and Guidance L21; 1999.

21 The Case Management Society. Code of ethics for case managers (available at www.cmsuk.org); 2007.

22 EEF. *Managing Sickness Absence: A Tool Kit for Changing Work Culture and Improving Business Performance* (available at www.eef.org.uk). London: EEF, 2007.

23 Stokes v. GKN (Nuts and Bolts) Ltd [1968] 1 WLR 1776.

24 Lewis J, Thornbory G. *Employment Law and Occupational Health: A Practical Handbook.* Oxford: Blackwell Publishing, 2006.

25 Health and Safety at Work etc. Act 1974, Section 2 (2) (a-e).

26 Greeen A, Youngs A. Occupational health – an over view of the legislation. In: Thornbory G, ed. *Occupational Health 2008: Making the Business Case – Special Report.* Cambridge: Workplace Law, 2007.

27 HSE. Work with Display Screen Equipment: Guidance on the Regulations, 2002.

28 Seedhouse D. *Health: The Foundations of Achievement*, 2nd edn. Chichester: John Wiley and Sons, 2001.

29 Roper N, Logan WW, Tierney AJ. *The Roper-Logan-Tierney Model of Nursing: Based on Activities of Living.* Edinburgh: Elsevier Health Sciences, 2000.

30 Information Commissioner. Employment Practices Code (available at www.ico.gov.uk); 2005.

31 Institute of Directors. *Wellbeing at Work: How to Manage Workplace Wellness to Boost Your Staff and Business Performance: A Directors Guide.* London: IOD, 2006.

32 Wright M, Marsden S. *Changing Business Behaviour*, CRR436/2002 (available at www.hse.gov.uk/research/crr_htm/2002/crr02436.htm); 2002.

33 CIPD. *Recruitment, Retention and Turnover, Annual Survey Report* (available at www.cipd.co.uk); 2007.

34 Chartered Institute of Personnel and Development. *Absence Management Annual Survey Report* (available at www.cipd.co.uk); 2008.

35 Kreis J, Bödeker W. *Health Related and Economic Benefits of Workplace Health Promotion and Prevention: Summary of Scientific Evidence* (available at www.enwhp.org/fileadmin/downloads/IGA-report_3_English.pdf). Essen: Buckbundesverband, 2004.

36 World Health Organization. Declaration of Workers Health (available at www.who.int/occupational_health/publications/declaration2006/en/index.html); 2006.

37 Donaldson L. *Smoke Free England – One Year On* (available at www.smokefreeengland.co.uk). London: DH, 2008.

38 Holford P, Nagle W, Kyne J, Rix D. Food for thought in occupational. *Health* 2008; **60**(6): 42-3.

39 Confederation of British Industry. *Absence and Labour Turnover Survey.* London: CBI/AXA, 2007.

Chapter 8

Occupational Health Nursing Practice

Greta Thornbory

Learning objectives

After reading this chapter you will be able to:

- Appreciate the role of the occupational health nurse (OHN) in the public health arena as defined by the NMC domains: search for health needs, awareness of health needs, influence on policies affecting health and facilitation of health-enhancing activities
- Appreciate the role of the OHN in advising and supporting the employer to employ a healthy and productive workforce
- Appreciate the role of the OHN in supporting and advising the worker from a health perspective, from commencement of employment to termination
- Discuss the professional, educational and managerial roles of the OHN from a public health perspective

Introduction

There is a long history of industrial or occupational health (OH) nursing dating back nearly 200 years, all of which is outlined in Irene Charley's book [1]. During those past times the link between health visiting and community nursing was acknowledged. It was realised as far back as the 1920s that there were substantial differences in the actual practice and therefore it was identified that the training and educational needs of the, then, industrial nurses needed separate consideration. Back in October 1932, a group of nurses held a meeting at the (Royal) College of Nursing to discuss the position of nurses in industry and discuss suitable training for them as they had identified that the proficiencies required in industry were beyond those covered by training in health visiting or district nursing, even though there were common areas among the three professions. The first course of training was offered in 1934 at the

(Royal) College of Nursing in conjunction with Bedford College for Women and was one academic year long. Since that time there have been great changes in industry, commence and technology and OH nurses (OHNs) have had to change their practice in line with the demands of the late twentieth- and early twenty-first-century business. This chapter aims to explore OH nursing practice in the twenty-first century to demonstrate how OH nursing fits into with the definitions of nursing given by both the International Council of Nurses (ICNs) and Royal College of Nursing (RCN) and the definitions of public health and public health nursing. It will also explore the role of OHNs against the NMC standards of proficiency for specialist community public health nurses (SCPHNs) and the RCN core competencies for OHNs.

Chapter 2 discussed the background to public health nursing and the various definitions of nursing. Here it is necessary to see how OH nursing fits into those definitions and how it fits into the principles of public health nursing outlined in Chapter 2 are utilised, these include:

- Promoting and protecting health
- Reducing risky behaviours and health equalities
- Preventing disease
- Assessing and monitoring the health of communities and populations to identify those at risk and those with health problems
- Assess priorities for action
- Collaborative working for health and well-being

These principles almost outline the role of the OHN as OH is all about protecting the health of the worker and promoting good health for the workforce; this has been explained in depth in Chapter 7. The main requirement of health and safety legislation is the assessment of risks to health and safety and putting in place suitable controls for the benefit of the workforce community and the wider community outside the workplace who may be affected. OHNs play an active part in advising management and employees about the risks to health and safety and ensuring that appropriate controls are in place, such as health surveillance, and preventing disease whether work related or not. All of this will be explained in more details later in the chapter.

Back in 2003, the Department of Health in conjunction with the RCN Society of OH Nursing produced a guide [2] for OHNs where it says that the workplace has enormous potential as a setting for improving the health of the adult population. This, of course, was nothing new to the OH nurse, although for some years the perception of public health meant that OH was not seen as part of the same agenda. Here it is identified that OHNs have access to a large number of people who are potentially at risk from adverse health effects caused by both work- and non-work-related health risks and who have established channels of communication in the workplace through which to deliver strategies for health promotion, protection and prevention. The document also said that with a public health perspective OHNs could identify the key issues for their workforce population by working as part of a multidisciplinary team irrespective of whether it is a large multinational, an SME or a specific type of industry. It goes on to say that for OHNs a public health approach is:

- Planning and delivering interventions and activities that are based on a systematic assessment of the health needs of the workforce that you are responsible for
- Working with others, including the workforce themselves, to agree what the priorities are and how they need to be addressed at individual and population levels
- Delivering health promotion and health protection programmes that are based on the best available evidence and evaluating their impact
- Working across professional and organisational boundaries, developing networks with others such as health visitors, practice nurses, GPs, infection control nurses, public health specialists, midwives and others in the NHS, local government, voluntary and business sectors

An example is shown in Case study 8.1.

Case Study 8.1 Hampshire county council (CC) OH service

In a modern-day occupational health service (OHS) practitioners need to be competent to deliver OH drivers based on:

- Organisational business need
- Government health strategy

This approach takes the focus away from absence management and illness, towards a more encompassing ethos and culture working towards attendance management, education and personal responsibility for good health.

Development of marketing materials such as booklets and advice leaflets need to be designed and published stating purpose, values and philosophy – the approach being to help staff to help themselves. Appropriate marketing will help sell services and demonstrate core messages such as the need to care for one's own health. An example of this is Hampshire CC OH 'schools pack' that gives a step-by-step guide to their biggest customer showing how best to utilise service provision, whilst the 'director pack' explains what we do and how we deliver to the other businesses.

Managing sickness absence can be a mine field and OH practitioners must be sure of their ground when giving advice. Up-to-date knowledge of health and safety and employment legislation is important as is an awareness of relevant case law, whilst clinical information gathered from clients needs to be accurate. Managing absence is a priority due to cost and it is essential to have sound strategies to help address the problem. At the same time the OH service needs to demonstrate added value by reducing the average clearance time on absence cases. Hampshire CC has managed to reduce this from around 20 days to 7 days. This means that the process for case management needs to be clearly defined. Client interviews need to be structured taking account of the time element and the quality of questions to be asked in order to bring specific answers.

It is best to put written information back to customers in a standard framework indicating:

- The main problem with health and work
- Any treatment that may affect work or delay progress
- Risk issues regarding the DDA
- Advice on a safe and timely return to work

Developing an intranet web page was essential to HCC marketing its services as it enabled a diverse range of products to be publicised.
Some examples are:

- The OH input into the policy health strategy
- Access to information and necessary OH documentation which can be downloaded
- Access to a plethora of up-to-date information on health topics and frequently asked questions
- Information on topical health issues
- Information on positive thinking and daily wellness habits emphasising the health and wellness element of OH

Working collaboratively on the 'service-level agreements' the OH service helps the customer understand a range of services that can realistically be delivered if we offer to bolt on, for example, three health seminars a year across the businesses. In practice this means that we are able to deliver what we say we can without putting the OHN under pressure. This also means that OH nurses have more variety in their job roles.

It became clear to HCC OH that on site health checks are a must in order to meet customer expectation, but when we offered these in 2007, we were overwhelmed by demand. Fortunately, these had been marketed as a trial so we were able to re-think the strategy. The next step is to tender for an online web-based health service that all 36,000 employees can access.

In terms of the day-to-day running of the department, we encourage a collaborative approach to case management, increasing our case reviews only for complex cases. As part of the case management process, we make an initial phone contact with the person who has referred the client before speaking to the client themselves; this enables OH to gauge the organisational viewpoint such as performance, attitude and ability.

A menu of educational workshops is offered to keep health issues on the agenda and OH is working with the safety teams and others to coordinate stress awareness, thus helping to identify any organisational issues and target health promotion.

Early on in the process areas of business with excessive absence were identified. Two OH advisers have been allocated to these businesses as the named person who will be able to offer an effective customer interface on a regular basis and to produce regular statistics as these are an all-important part of this process. This will be regularly reviewed and evaluated.

In the previous chapter the people that go to make up the OH team was explained in detail, here we can see that OHNs will have to work with the even wider health team outside of their particular place of work. Indeed this concept of collaboration is one in line with the NMC principles in the standards of proficiency [3].

Of course, not all UK employees are working on home shores. Many people are employed and work for international companies or are sent by their employers to undertake work in foreign, often hostile climes; examples of these are the news journalists and camera crews, non-governmental organisations such as the Red Cross and Save the Children, the armed forces and research scientists. Yet, as UK citizens they and their employers are governed by UK laws and so consideration must be given to their health and well-being whilst at work; their public health remains a concern and OHNs must be able to help and advise those people. In Case study 8.1, one OHN gives an example of the work her company must consider.

Case Study 8.2   The UK Employee abroad

Providing global OHS for the oil and gas industry and any other commercial or industrial services provides many challenges, with public health being a major consideration. The three elements to public health are infrastructure, disease profile and workplace environment.

Infrastructure
Working in remote locations and in developing countries, where the infrastructure is not always conducive to the maintenance of public health, the OHN has to assess and advise on both the workplace and the local health risks. The main issues are:

- *Local health care provision* – how to access quality care and access resources; the limited monitoring of ill health from a distance with subsequent education and preventative service.

- *Water quality*, often contaminated due to old pipe work or the use of well water, access to potable water for remote or offshore situations and managing water supplies in company residences. One of the main issues is the mineralisation of water resulting in kidney dysfunction, urolithiasis and other calculi and the risk from legionella or other bacteria.
- *Food quality* is primarily affected by spoilage which is common in hot countries, pests and food safety. Although there are international standards for personal hygiene and food hygiene they are not always in place and working effectively.
- *Waste management* in remote locations and developing countries is usually via septic tanks. Food wastes are sometimes stored ready for collection and attract vermin. Biohazard waste is not always segregated or managed to European standards with appropriate sharps boxes and incineration.

Disease profile

Using the WHO research and data provides a baseline to assess the burden of disease for the specific countries. The main issues are:

- Water and vector-borne disease from malaria to haemorrhagic fever and rabies
- Other infectious disease including scabies (associated with cramped living conditions), influenza and gastrointestinal disease associated with poor personal and food hygiene practices
- Travel-related conditions such as isolation and sexual and reproductive health also count towards the disease profile
- Mortality and morbidity due to lifestyle, age and genetic factor, as well as health beliefs

Environment

- Extremes of temperature not only have a physical and psychological impact they also affect the ability to exercise and socialise outdoors
- Air quality can be affected by pollution and industrial by-products, which may be controlled if within your own company but not so easily if it is from a neighbouring company
- Industrial pollution also includes noise, odours and chemical

Therefore, organisations commission a health impact assessment to identify the significant public health issues whilst the companies work both internally and with external partners and government organisations to control the associated risk to health, which is where the OHN plays a vital role. The OHN has to ensure that his or her advice, support and service delivery are in line with the public health constraints and support the improvements required.

Christina Butterworth, Health Risk Manager, BG Group

The role of the OHN

The role of the OHN is complex and covers many different aspects and disciplines of nursing. Whitaker and Baranski [4] give the following list:

- Clinician
- Specialist
- Manager
- Coordinator
- Adviser
- Health educator
- Counsellor
- Researcher

This is a long list of different roles for one person and many nurses working in OH may well not be equipped with all those skills.

> ### Activity 8.1
>
> Consider your work in OH and write a brief paragraph on how you fulfil each of the roles outlined above.

A public health approach means working with both populations and individuals [2], certainly from the perspective of competence in those areas then basic nurse training will not have equipped the OHN. The RCN has produced a list of 'competencies' for OH nursing [5] and graded the nurse into three distinct categories of competent, experienced and expert OHN – see Box 8.1 – this was produced to be in line with the Department of Health Agenda for change knowledge and skills framework [6].

> ### Box 8.1 OH nursing-level descriptors
>
> **Competent OHN**
>
> - First-level registered nurse
> - Two years post-basic experience
> - Post-basic education and training equivalent to university diploma
> - Works under guidance of established protocols and procedures at operational level
> - Maintains safe and competent practice
>
> **Experienced OHN**
>
> - Two years experience in OH setting
> - Post-basic education and training equivalent to university degree
> - Holds or working towards a recordable/registered OHN qualification with the NMC

- Develops and establishes protocols and procedures at operational level
- Develops and leads on safe and competent practice

Expert OHN

- Five years experience in OH setting
- Post-basic education and training equivalent to university higher degree
- Holds a recordable/registered OHN qualification with the NMC
- Develops, leads and establishes protocols and procedures at operational and strategic levels
- Innovates, develops and leads on safe and competent practice
- Leads and develops consultant occupational nursing and consultancy

Adapted from RCN Competencies 2005.

Even though OHNs work outside the NHS many private employers base their pay scales on those of the NHS, although it has to be said that they are under no obligation to offer the same pay and conditions as the NHS and many do not. It was hoped that these competencies would enable employers to see the scope and value of OHNs as well as to help with determining their pay scale; however, personal communication has indicated that they have not been found to be of any real use to private employers.

The RCN Competencies have also been mapped against the NMC standards for SCPHN to show how the work of the OHN fits into the NMC requirements. The RCN competency framework lists 12 sections where the OHN needs to be competent to practice at one or other of the 3 levels:

(1) Self-assessment
(2) Core transferable skills
(3) Core leadership and management skills
(4) Core quality assurance and research skills
(5) Legal and ethical issues
(6) Risk assessment
(7) Heath promotion, protection and surveillance
(8) Sickness, absence and rehabilitation
(9) Psychological and psychosocial interventions
(10) Ergonomics
(11) Occupational hygiene
(12) Maintaining safety and accident control

So, between the different roles outlined by Whitaker and Baranski, the RCN level descriptors and competencies and the NMC principles it is not surprising that many people get lost when trying to find out exactly what an OHN does! Indeed the wide variation in the OH nurse's role that can be observed in different industries reflects different demands and priorities from within those different settings, but also different stages in the development of the OHS. In some settings the role is defined more narrowly within a commercial contract for services that makes explicit that the employer will pay for only those services that they want to purchase. In this case the role of the OH nurse may be seen only within the context of enabling the employer to comply with his legal duties. In other settings the role is much wider and can encompass many different types of activities with different, often complementary, benefits. It is perhaps easier to consider the role of the OHN with each stage of employment. The employer must consider the health of the worker from the time they are employed until the time they leave employment and beyond. So let us now consider the role of the OHN at each stage of the employment process.

Pre-employment and recruitment

Employing people is a risky and costly process; on average in 2008, recruitment costs £4667 per employee [7]. It could be said that employers only want to employ healthy or fit people because they will give better service, but then we know that defining health and fitness is not easy [8]. Involving the OH service, and in particular the OHN, from an early stage in recruitment is advisable. To start with the OH service can advise companies on the health aspects of their recruitment policies and procedures, particularly where risk assessments indicate that there is a particular hazard in the working environment which could affect the health of employees. The OHN cannot do this unless they have knowledge and understanding of the workplace, the type of work and the job demands and the skills to assess risks and make recommendations.

It is not in nursing and medical training to know the ins and outs of factories, work processes and the many different types of employment, some of which are extremely hazardous. Where practical the OHN should visit the working environment where he or she is employed, to gain knowledge and information of the different jobs and work processes that the organisation undertakes and to get to know the various managers, as well as employees and staff and/or trade union representatives. Only then can the OHN give an informed opinion on the fitness needs for different jobs. Where there are specific hazards and demands advice may be needed from other members of the OH team, such as the OH Physician, ergonomist, safety officer or occupational hygienist. Some types of work may have either statutory or mandatory health requirements, e.g. working with tools that may cause hand arm vibration (HAVs), working with specific substances such as asbestos or lead, and these will need to be considered.

Once management have completed the risk assessment and the health requirements for the job based on that assessment have been discussed and agreed with the OH service, then together they will be able to lay down some health criteria. There has been little research into pre-employment health assessment; however, research that has been undertaken shows that there is little value, either in financial terms or health terms, in extensive pre-employment health assessment unless there is a specific health needs for the job [9]. This research undertaken in the early 1990s demonstrated that 98% of applicants were found 'fit for work' using a self-administered questionnaire followed by an interview by a nurse. The conclusion was that pre-employment health assessment had its limitations in terms of its ability to detect clinical conditions and to predict the health status of employees once in employment; no subsequent research has challenged this statement.

Another OH audit [10] undertaken for two years, April 2003 to April 2005, where 4482 pre-employment forms were scrutinised no one was refused employment for health reasons. According to the audit the estimated costs of scrutinising pre-employment health declaration forms amounted to 15 minutes per form and almost the cost of one full-time OH adviser at a salary of circa £30 000 pa. This sum was reached by adding up the time it takes to:

- Scrutinise each form
- To clarify statements and get correct information
- Complete the necessary records and documentation
- Return the documentation and answer any queries

Further research into pre-employment questionnaires was undertaken in 2006 by Ballard [11]. He also highlighted the time-consuming aspects of this function concurring with Hargreaves' findings above. He concluded that not everyone agrees that the effectiveness of pre-employment health assessment justifies the time and resources invested in it.

According to the Chartered Institute of Personnel and Development (CIPD) [7] survey, 25% of organisations had refused employment to people who had lied on their applications. In her article on honesty and knowledge at pre-employment, Kloss [12] says that there is no duty on a prospective employee to declare a health condition; however, if he or she makes a deliberate lie then they may be acting unlawfully; as yet there is no legal precedent. So all this does not augur well for pre-employment health assessment being of any particular value in the long term of either saving money or predicting the health outcomes of prospective employees.

The Data Protection Act Employment Code of Practice [13] says that only necessary information should be obtained and kept on individuals, so employers and OH services can only ask for information from employees that is necessary and that includes health information.

Activity 8.2

Review your pre-employment procedures and find out when the last audit of your records system was undertaken. Consider if any changes need to be made in your area of practice and what contribution you can make to bring about those changes

Disability and work

The implications of the Disability Discrimination Act (DDA) mean that one cannot turn down applicants who have a health condition unless due consideration has been to making 'reasonable adjustments' to the job and the workplace. One point to note here is that there is help and support from the government department, the Department of Work and Pensions (DWP) through their Access to Work scheme and the specialist advisers and the Disability Employment Advisers (DEAs). The DEA will help to provide specialist support to people who are recently disabled, or those whose disability or health condition has deteriorated and who need employment advice. They provide support to disabled people who are having difficulty in getting a job because of their disability, and also to employed people who are concerned about losing their job because of a disability whilst the Access to Work advisers provide support to disabled people and their employers to help overcome work-related obstacles resulting from a disability.

Pre-employment health assessment today

Hargreaves [10] trialled a new approach to pre-employment health and it is proving attractive in several organisations. Recommendations from the trial are that pre-employment health assessments should continue where the risk assessment has identified that there are health and safety issues or safety critical standards to be met such as for health care workers, construction workers or drivers who need to meet the Driver and Vehicle Licensing Agency standards etc. The suggestion is that pre-employment health assessment is eliminated for the majority of workers and the following three questions be incorporated into the recruitment form and assessed by Human Resources (HR) personnel:

- Do you need any special aids/adaptations to assist you at work, whether or not you have a disability?
- Are you having, or waiting for, treatment or investigations of any kind at present?
- Have you ever had any health problems which may have been caused or made worse by work?
  - Answer YES to any one of the questions and the candidate must be referred to OH for assessment
  - Answer NO to all questions and accept as fit for employment

This would mean that HR/Personnel are aware at the recruitment stage that the DDA may apply, or that there is a health problem to be considered as only prospective employees who have answered yes to any one or more of the questions would be seen for a thorough confidential assessment by the OH professionals, usually an OH nurse in the first instance who may refer the person to the OH physician depending on their case history. However, more research is needed to develop an evidence base for pre-employment health assessment.

Of course where there are specific hazards in the job, or there are statutory or mandatory health surveillance requirements on-employment health assessments or even a medical examination by an OH physician maybe necessary, e.g., for divers, airline pilots etc. but as Smedley et al. [14] say the rationale for the fitness assessment should be clear to all parties.

Records

Once a person is employed then his or her OH record, or medical record, is created and this should contain only health details that relate directly to what is needed for that specific post/job. This record remains a confidential record to the OH team [15].

A survey undertaken by Ballard [11] revealed that some OH services enquired about 160 different conditions, symptoms or syndromes. This is excessive and, according to the DPA, no personal information should be obtained or kept unless it is relevant to the job; there seems to be no evidence base for obtaining and keeping such details. Asking about such things as 'family history' is not really relevant with regards to being fit for work and has no place on OH.

Regular auditing of the OH service is recommended [16, 17] and the Information Commissioner recommends a regular audit or 'impact assessment' of the collection and storage used for the OH records system to ensure that the collection of health information does actually address the risks it is directed at. The DPA Employment CoP gives clear guidelines for this.

It must be remembered that employee OH records are confidential and where health surveillance is required by law then two different types of records will be generated:

(1) *The OH record*: This is the confidential document held securely by the OH service/department and is the clinical record of the employee relevant to his or her job and visits to the OH service. It is not available to anyone outside of the OH service other than the employee to whom it relates without the informed written consent of that employee. It should be kept whilst the employee continues in that employment and it is suggested that they are kept for a period of time after employment ceases. There is no statutory requirement to keep them, but sickness records and medical reports should be kept for 3 years and accident and injury records should be kept up to 12 years after the end of employment. These latter records may be held by HR/Personnel as they are not the clinical OH record.

(2) *The health record*: This is a record of health surveillance results, i.e. that the employee is fit to continue his or her work following whatever health surveillance procedures have been undertaken. More details on health records will be given in the section on health surveillance.

OHNs should follow the guidance given by the NMC on record keeping [19]. There is a section on the ownership of records which relates specifically to OH nursing and OH records.

Report writing

The OHNs will be expected to write reports for employers in several circumstances, e.g. assessment on employment, sickness absence referral or a workplace assessment. It is easier if the OH department has a procedure agreed with management and prepared a template or pro forma to be used both for the referral and the report. This avoids all confusion on both sides. It also enables the employee to give his or her written consent to disclosure which is required as doctors and nurses have a duty of care to maintain patient/client information as confidential.

Confidentiality

This is enshrined in the relevant professional codes of practice [20] and reinforced with the DPA and Section 4 of the DPA Employment Code. However, when it comes to giving reports to management OHNs often come into conflict. As Butterworth [21] says 'We need to say less often *"I cannot tell you, it is confidential"* and to say more often *"I can see why you would want that information, but I have a duty of care to my patient/client. However, I would like to work with you on what sort of reasonable adjustments we can put into place"'*. In other words, be positive and not negative and where possible get the patient/clients written consent to disclose – if not everything then at least some aspects of his or her case. Again, it helps if the OH service has a template or pro forma for the employee to sign for such disclosures.

When writing medical reports individuals have a right of access to that report under the Access to Medical Reports Act 1988 (AMRA). Although the Act says specifically that medical reports relate to reports prepared by a medical practitioner who is or has been responsible for the clinical care of the individual, it is generally accepted that OH health professionals would probably fall into this category although there has been no case law under this Act to test this. Suffice it to say the DPA allows individuals the right to access to their records.

> ### Activity 8.3
>
> Before reading the next section write notes on what you understand health surveillance is all about and then compare your notes with the text below.

Health surveillance

The Management of Health and Safety at Work Regulations not only require employers to make a suitable and sufficient assessment of the risks to health and safety at work, but also under Regulation 6, they require every employer to provide health surveillance appropriate to those risks identified by the assessment. Risk assessment is the first step to deciding whether or not health surveillance is needed within an organisation or changed. It is important to remember that health surveillance should not be used for any other reason without specific permission of the individual. Employers who seek to check to see if someone is under the influence of alcohol or drugs or has a disease caused by a blood-borne virus transmitted by sexual means could be construed as in breach of the Human Rights Act, unless there is a specific need identified by the risk assessment in that particular employment.

The Health and Safety Executive (HSE) [22] defines health surveillance as:

Putting in place systematic, regular and appropriate procedures to detect early signs of work-related ill health among employees exposed to certain health risks; and acting on the results.

HSE go on to outline the benefits of health surveillance as:

- Providing information to detect harmful health effects at an early stage, thereby protecting employees and confirming whether they are still fit to do their jobs
- Checking control measures and giving feedback on risk assessments
- Providing data, by means of health records, to detect and evaluate risks
- Providing an opportunity to train and instruct employees further in safe and healthy working practices
- Giving employees an opportunity to raise concerns about the effect of work on health

Types of health surveillance

There are many different types of health surveillance depending on the hazard and how it affects the human body. So it is important to make sure that whatever procedures or 'screening' is carried out fulfils the criteria laid down by recognised bodies; otherwise OH professionals may be in breach of their ethical codes of practice. Screening in medicine is a strategy used to identify disease and its intention is to identify disease in a given community early, thus enabling earlier intervention and management in the hope to reduce mortality and suffering from a disease. However, not all screening tests have been shown to benefit the person being screened; overdiagnosis, misdiagnosis and creating a false sense of security are some of the potential adverse effects of screening. The basic principles of screening were laid down in 1968 by Wilson and Junger and adopted by the World Health Organization [23] as follows:

- The condition should be an important health problem
- There should be a treatment for the condition
- Facilities for diagnosis and treatment should be available
- There should be a latent stage of the disease
- There should be a test or examination for the condition

- The test should be acceptable to the population
- The natural history of the disease should be adequately understood
- There should be an agreed policy on who to treat
- The total cost of finding a case should be economically balanced in relation to medical expenditure as a whole
- Case finding should be a continuous process, not just a 'once and for all' project

Subsequently, these criteria have been updated and expanded by the UK National Screening Committee (www.nsc.nhs.uk/pdfs/criteria.pdf). So no health surveillance or 'screening' procedures should be undertaken just for the sake of it. There is no point in carrying out an invasive procedure, such as obtaining a blood test, then telling the person there is a problem but have no means of treating it. It is not always necessary for health surveillance to involve the services of OH professionals and certain surveillance can be undertaken by either responsible persons or even other qualified persons as outlined in Chapter 7.

Certain critical professions produce guidelines on their health surveillance requirements, e.g. for drivers (www.dvla.gov.uk/medical/about_dri_med.aspx) or the UK Civil Aviation Authority (CAA) (www.caa.co.uk). Because of the recent age discrimination legislation [24] many of these are now all under review as, at present, different health surveillance procedures are required according to age. This could be seen as discriminatory and consideration must be given to the evidence base for separate health surveillance for different groups. In the HSE guidance on health surveillance they state that these legal duties of assessing fitness to work should not be confused with health surveillance. On the other hand, they are all part of the 'watching over' brief to protect the worker and others; so whether or not they are part of 'health surveillance' really falls to semantics!

Screening 'procedures'

This section aims to explain the different types of screening procedures that can be undertaken as part of health surveillance. It is not intended to cover absolutely all screening procedures used in health surveillance but will cover those most commonly used.

Questionnaires

Using a questionnaire is a screening procedure under health surveillance and may be used with a number of different hazards. The design is important as are the procedures for administering the questionnaire. Confidentiality must be maintained and no questions asked which are not specifically related to the particular hazard and its effects. It should be checked by a suitably qualified person, such as an OH nurse, who will be able to take the appropriate action if necessary.

Skin surveillance

Occupational skin disease is a common OH problem. It is due to either irritation or sensitisation and causes dermatitis. A number of occupations where substances are handled can cause problems [25]. Skin surveillance is one of the simplest forms of health surveillance where an employee may undertake the checks for himself, he or she will need to be properly informed and trained about the signs and symptoms of any skin conditions that may arise from his or her work and where to go for further advice. Self-assessment on its own is not sufficient without complementary checks undertaken by a specifically trained person and the whole programme supervised by OH professionals.

Respiratory surveillance

There are a number of substances that are known to affect the respiratory system and may cause occupational asthma. Guidelines for the health surveillance of people exposed to respiratory sensitisers and respiratory irritants has been produced by the British Occupational Health Research Foundation (BOHRF) [26] and supported by the HSE. There is also ongoing research in this field, where a risk of occupational asthma is identified, the surveillance commences with a respiratory questionnaire on employment and is then completed annually, although during the first two years of employment this would be more frequent. Such a questionnaire would be designed and scrutinised by OH professionals and would include:

- Type and duration, frequency and intensity of exposure to the sensitiser over a given period
- Any changes in signs and symptoms, such sore eyes or a runny nose not linked to a cold or flu
- Any respiratory signs or symptoms, such as a wheeze, shortness of breath or any difficulty in breathing, coughs or tickly throat that have developed since the last questionnaire completed

The results are then logged onto the employee's health record. When a problem is identified there may be a need for further investigations such as skin-prick testing and blood sampling or lung function tests. These screening tests must be undertaken by appropriately qualified people, not necessarily a doctor or nurse, but someone who has received training in the necessary technical skills, such as an OH technician. However, the results must be viewed and interpreted by an OH or respiratory health professional.

Blood testing

It is a legal requirement for certain types of workers, such as lead workers, health care workers and critical safety workers to have blood tested. Lead workers require a blood test to ascertain that the environmental controls in the workplace are effective and also that certain workplace personal hygiene procedures are being adhered to. This is the opposite to the health surveillance by blood test of people working in safety critical areas who may require blood screening to ascertain that they have not used drugs or alcohol, although there are other, less invasive, tests that can be done, such as hair sampling and urine testing which would better fulfil the screening criteria. Health care workers require blood testing to check immunity following immunisation against certain work-related conditions such as hepatitis B. Other blood tests may also be required to confirm if sensitivity to a skin or respiratory irritant is suspected. However, venepuncture is an invasive procedure and should be avoided unless absolutely necessary and that there is no alternative effective method of surveillance.

Eyesight testing

It will depend on the reason for the eyesight testing as to which method of testing is used. A professionally qualified optician or optometrist is necessary to carry out a full eye test and it may be advisable for a baseline test to be carried out when employing people in jobs with specific visual requirements. However, there are machines that can be purchased which will test for specific work requirements, such as for display screen equipment use with computers and depth perception for forklift truck drivers. It is best to discuss this with an OH adviser to ensure that the correct vision testing is undertaken. The simple vision test is the Snellen Chart which provides a standardised test of visual acuity. As well as visual acuity details on the other tests that may be necessary, such as colour testing for certain jobs, then the HSE guide for employers on colour vision examination gives comprehensive details [27].

Audiometry

Audiometry is undertaken at the workplace where it is required to check the effectiveness of the noise control measures. It became mandatory at intervals of three years (sometimes more often) for all UK employees exposed to levels of 85 dB(A) on a daily basis and those exposed to peak sound pressure levels above 137 dB [28]. However, audiometry is only part of a hearing conservation programme and the HSE say that as a minimum, a programme of health surveillance should include:

- Audiometric testing (baseline assessment on first entering a job involving noise exposure, annual testing for two years, then three yearly testing)
- Arrangements to receive medical advice on management of affected employees
- Arrangements to receive anonymised information to demonstrate effectiveness of controls

Training to use audiometry equipment is usually available from the manufactures of the equipment and may be undertaken by suitably qualified people such as OH technicians.

Health records

Any form of health surveillance requires a record to be kept. They are different from a clinical or medical record and the two should not be confused. Health surveillance records are kept as an historical record of exposure to the hazardous process or procedure; as a record of the outcome of health surveillance procedures in terms of fitness to work, restrictions etc. and they provide information for the statutory bodies to show health surveillance has been undertaken.

Health surveillance and health records must contain:

- Full name
- Date of birth
- Sex
- Permanent address
- National insurance number
- Date of commencement of present job
- An historical record of exposure to the hazard for which health surveillance is required
- The conclusions of any health surveillance procedures, i.e. fit to work; fit to work subject to certain conditions etc. The date and by whom they were carried out

Retention of health records

Health records should be kept as long as the person is under health surveillance. However, there are certain statutory requirements to keep health records for much longer, some for up to 50 years, so it is important to check the relevant legislation and guidance notes or codes of practice published by the HSE.

Case Study 8.3

Lotus cars has its own in-house OH department of a full-time OHN and part-time OH technician. The team is led by the OH and safety manager who is a qualified SCPHN in OH and who contracts in the services of an OH physician, physiotherapists and a counsellor.

The company specialises in the design and build of elite sports cars and the provision of engineering consultancy services both in the UK and overseas. It employs a workforce of approximately 1000 staff and approximately 50% will be working within areas that require some degree of health surveillance.

A large proportion of the working week is dedicated to the health surveillance process with clinical assessments, follow-ups, workplace visits and report writing and documentation. By providing an in-house service, we are able to review any identified OH problems both quickly and efficiently and are able to act promptly. We work proactively with both health and safety and managerial staff by looking at the source of the matter and aim to prevent work-related ill health rather than reactively attempting to cure and control the problem.

The OH team is familiar with the workforce and the working environment and is able to address the matter of sickness absence efficiently by close working relationships with HR, line management and employees alike. This close relationship has resulted in sickness absence levels of approximately 2%, far below the considered national average and one that we are proud to have achieved.

Other considerations for monitoring health at work

Business travel health

Employees who travel overseas as part of their role, or who may work for long periods overseas for UK companies are still covered by UK health and safety legislation. Therefore the employer has a duty of care and should make sure that a risk assessment is carried out and that the risks to health are addressed before travel. OH services are involved in offering such advice and in many cases providing suitable immunisation programmes, information and training sessions.

Night workers

Night workers are entitled to a free health assessment before they start working nights and on a regular basis while they are working nights according to the Working Time Regulations 1998. In many cases it will be appropriate to do this once a year, though employers can offer a health assessment more than once a year if they feel it is necessary. Workers do not have to take the opportunity to have a health assessment (but it must be offered by the employer). A health assessment can be made up of two parts: a questionnaire and a medical examination. The latter is only necessary if the employer has doubts about the worker's fitness for night work.

New and expectant mothers

New and expectant mothers are required under the Management of Health and Safety at Work Regulations to have a separate risk assessment undertaken for them in order to ensure that their work does not affect them or the unborn child.

Managing absence, disability and rehabilitation

Managing absence is a management responsibility but OH services can do a lot to help and support employers in effectively managing absence. When

Table 8.1 Reasons for absence from work.

Planned	Unplanned
Annual leave	Military service
Study leave	Jury service
Maternity/paternity	Bereavement/compassionate leave
Time off in lieu	Unplanned health problems
Sabbatical/break in service	
Planned health care	

talking about absence most people think solely of sickness absence but there are many other reasons for people being absent from work and these fall into two main categories – planned and unplanned (see Table 8.1).

These are mostly planned absences and so management accommodates them; even some sickness absence can be planned, such as routine surgery. Problems occur when employees take unplanned sick leave and the biggest cost to employers occurs with short-term minor illness, generally regarded as less than four weeks, but the majority of which is less than seven days.

Two organisations undertake annual business absence surveys, the Confederation of British Industries (CBI) in conjunction with AXA [29] and the CIPD [30]. Other, work-related absence statistics are published regularly by the HSE (www.hse.gov.uk/statistics/index.htm). The interesting factors from these surveys indicate that despite initiatives sickness absence, particularly in the public sector, is not reducing and that 12% of sickness absence is thought not to be genuine and is used to extend weekends, for special events such as birthdays and for important football matches, with many people taking time off sick to deal with home and family responsibilities. Whitaker [31] says that there are a number of different perspectives from which sickness absence can be viewed and Table 8.2 shows the factors that have been linked to increase rates of sickness absence.

Both surveys highlight those aspects of sickness absence management which work well. What remains a constant are the reasons for long-term absence, i.e. over four weeks; these are musculoskeletal disorders and mental ill health related to stress, anxiety and depression. It is especially in these areas that OH can play a part in supporting management with rehabilitation advice.

Principles of sickness absence management

Develop policies and procedures

The initial key to sound absence management is the policies and procedures developed by management. They should be clearly defined, commonly understood and widely accepted [32]. All stakeholders, including the OH service, need to be involved in the development of such policies and procedures and

Table 8.2 Factors that can affect sickness absence.

Macro level	Organisational level	Individual level
Climate	Nature of the industry	Age
Epidemics	Working conditions	Gender
Provision of health	Job demands	Occupational status
care services	Size of the enterprise	Job satisfaction
Social insurance	Characteristics of the	Length of service
systems	workforce	Personality
Sickness	Workforce availability	Life crises
certification	Industrial relations	Family
practices	Supervisory quality	responsibility
Taxation	Personnel policies	Social support
Pensionable age	Labour turnover	Leisure activities
Social attitudes	The provision of OH	The health status of
Economic climate	services	the individual
Available		Alcohol intake
alternative		
employment		
or		
unemployment		

From Whitaker [31] with permission.

rehabilitation should be included as part of the overall absence management policy and procedures.

Return to work procedures

Return to work interviews (RTWI) by line managers, trigger mechanisms and the use of disciplinary procedures were rated as the most effective approaches to deal with short-term absence in both surveys. For some years now, according to the surveys, RTWI appear to be more effective than disciplinary measures and the recommendations are that it should be carried out by the (appropriately trained) line manager after every period of unscheduled absence.

After RTWI, trigger mechanisms, e.g. ten or more days off sick, indicate that the involvement of OH services is needed along with introducing rehabilitation programmes. According to the CIPD survey, involvement of OH is key to managing long-term absence. ACAS [33] say it is also important to keep in touch with employees through regular contact when they are on long-term sick leave. The last few years has seen a substantial increase in the number of employers developing employee well-being programmes as an effective means of reducing the cost of absence [34].

The aim of the RTWI is that the employee will find it easier to return to work. However, RTW is still a big step which causes anxiety and exacerbates all sorts of health implications, so a phased return to work is often suggested as well as the assessment of whether any reasonable adjustments are needed.

The stigma attached to any sort of mental illness, which stress-related conditions are, needs careful handling. Employers, HR and managers should be aware of the resources available, e.g. the Mindful Employer (www. mindfulemployer.net) initiative which is aimed at increasing awareness of mental health at work and providing support for businesses in recruiting and retaining staff.

Referral to OH for help and advice on long-term absence cases must be a formal procedure and not seen as a threat or disciplinary measure. Such behaviour undermines the professional and confidential nature of an OH service. OH professionals are also frustrated by the person who turns up to the department saying they have been sent by management without any formal referral. This is why the referral process must be included in the policy and procedures and it is better to use a pro forma. Any form of referral should be written and then signed by the referring manager and the employee with a statement that the reason for referral has been explained and that he or she consents to an OH report being prepared as per the Data Protection Act and the employee's rights under this Act.

Once the OH service has received the referral form, they can then make the necessary arrangements to see the employee and, where necessary, obtain further details and make recommendations by writing a report to whoever made the request. Further details may be required from the employee's doctor, particularly a specialist. Caution should be taken when requesting reports from GPs as it is believed that these do not generally make a difference to the OH decision [35]. Obtaining further details is not cheap; doctors, both GPs and specialists, require professional fees for preparing and sending a report to an employer, even if it is through the OH service. It is best to find out the cost, by telephone if necessary before requesting. There is a saving to the company money in the long run if the correct approach is taken and the employee returned to work.

Principles of rehabilitation and case management

'Rehabilitation is not about forcing people back to work. Work, in fact, is often a crucial step in helping people return to health. And businesses have much to gain in terms of reduced sickness absence, and improved staff engagement and retention', so Lord McKenzie from Department of Work and Pension said in July 2007 at the launch of a new 'vocational rehabilitation' taskforce. Waddell and Burton [36] say that many people do and can work with health problems. Well-designed clinical and occupational management should minimise the impact on work performance and productivity; timing for rehabilitation is critical and there are many harmful effects of staying away from work for too long.

Vocational rehabilitation is defined as:

a process which enables people with functional, psychological, developmental, cognitive and emotional impairments or health conditions to overcome barriers to accessing, maintaining or returning to employment or other useful occupation [37].

Traditionally, the UK health services have concentrated on the three tiers of health care: primary, secondary and tertiary which is rehabilitation. Waddell and Burton have demonstrated [38] that work is good for your health and can be an effective part of health care, especially if used in the first to sixth month of absence. They show that unemployment is strongly associated with poor mental and physical health, higher mortality, higher medical and hospital needs and low self-esteem.

The new standards published by the Vocational Rehabilitation Association (VRA) [36] say that the rehabilitation process is interdisciplinary by nature, and may require functional, biopsychosocial, behavioural and/or vocational interventions. They go on to list the techniques required, but not limited to as:

- Assessment and appraisal
- Goal setting and intervention planning
- Provision of health advice and promotion, in support of returning to work
- Support for self-management of health conditions
- Career (vocational) counselling
- Individual and group counselling focused on facilitating adjustments to the medical and psychosocial impact of disability
- Case management, referral and service coordination
- Programme evaluation and research
- Interventions to remove environmental, employment and attitudinal obstacles
- Consultation services among multiple parties and regulatory systems
- Job analysis, job development and placement services, including assistance with employment
- Job accommodations
- The provision of consultation about and access to rehabilitation technology

These required appropriately trained and skilled people to deal with them and the VRA standards go on to lay down standards for practice in this area. OH professionals should be able to fulfil these criteria with the help and support of other VR professionals.

The use of case managers is regarded as useful for rehabilitation; the Case Management Society UK (www.cmsuk.org) says that the role of a case manager is to work with clients on an individual basis. They define case management as:

A collaborative process which assesses, plans, implements, co-ordinates, monitors and evaluates the options and services required to meet an individuals health, care, educational and employment needs, using communication and available resources to promote quality cost effective outcomes.

This sounds very much like the 'nursing process' and here rehabilitation requires the OHN to work within a multidisciplinary team using a biopsychosocial model [35]. This model considers the biological or physical/mental health condition together with the psychological/personal factors which influence the functioning of the individual and the social contexts and pressures on behaviour and functioning as explained in Chapter 2. Therefore, role of OH in the rehabilitation of employees is to:

- Assess the individual by identifying the health problem and obtaining further medical information if necessary
- Assess their workplace and possibly undertake or obtain a job analysis or risk assessment
- Assess the employee's ability to get to and from, in and out of work, particularly in emergencies
- Arranging ongoing treatment such as psychological or physical therapies where necessary
- Advising management, by means of a written report, on reasonable adjustments or restrictive duties where necessary

Tolley [39] makes recommendations for graduated or structured return to work:

- Reduction of hours per day but not less than four hours per day
- Working from home or carrying out partial duties
- Gradually increase hours/days over a period of 6–8 weeks maximum
- Therapeutic interventions should take place outside of these shorter working hours
- OH service to review the progress on a regular basis

In the first instance it may be worth recommending that the long-term absent employee returning for coffee, tea or lunch with his or her colleagues to break the ice.

There are a number of initiatives being planned by government departments aimed at helping to improve the peoples return to work following sickness absence, particularly with regard to the GPs 'sick note'. It has been suggested that GPs should consider more what people are able to do rather than what they cannot do [40]. Pilot studies will be undertaken in the UK before these will be introduced and at this stage there is no news on this topic.

Case Study 8.4

Neylon Occupational Health Limited (NOHL) is a nurse-led service. It covers the full spectrum of OH from office-based firms to the manufacturing and construction industries. NOHL provides a service in line with evolving standards and practice within the field of OH which incorporates health surveillance, sickness/absence with the focus on rehabilitation, health assessments, drugs and alcohol testing, health promotion, travel health, management referrals, physiotherapy, first-aid training, manual handling.

I also provide seminars to GPs, OH physicians and other professionals to move the focus from absence to work and rehabilitation. NOHL is a small provider but has the added advantage of being able to provide a bespoke provision to its clients ensuring continuity and a personalised service. The main disadvantage to me, as a nurse-led provider, is the degree of responsibility and the lack of professional support as a lone practitioner. The best way to counteract this is to continue to update my skills, attend conferences and seminars and attend OH professional membership groups.

Sandra Neylon

Summary

It can be seen that the role of the OH service and in particular the role of the OHN in the protection and promotion of worker's health is key to a public health nursing role. This is clearly illustrated in the case studies and Case study 8.4 demonstrates that this can be achieved through small as well as large businesses. The community of workers has long been on the fringes of health care provision in the UK; now that it is clearly seen as part of public health and is vital for the health of the population and the UK economy there are initiatives being discussed at national levels [41] to raise the profile of OH even higher. It is, therefore, essential for OHNs to keep up to date with their CPD and what is happening in this important health care speciality.

References

1 Charley I. *The Birth of Industrial Nursing*. London: Ballière, Tindall and Cox, 1954.
2 DH. *Taking a Public Health Approach in the Workplace*. London: DH, 2003.
3 Nursing and Midwifery Council. *Standards of Proficiency for Specialist Community Public Health Nurses*. London: NMC, 2004.
4 Whitaker S, Baranski B. *The Role of the Occupational Health Nurse in Workplace Health Management*. Bilthoven: WHO, 2001.
5 RCN. *Competencies: An Integrated Career and Competency Framework for Occupational Health Nursing*. London: RCN, 2005.
6 Department of Health. *NHS Knowledge and Skills Framework (NHS KSF) and the Development and Review Process*. London: DH, 2004.
7 Chartered Institute of Personnel and Development. *Recruitment, Retention and Turnover: Annual Survey Report 2008*. London: CIPD, 2008.

8 Seedhouse D. *Health: The Foundations of Achievement*, 2nd edn. Chichester: John Wiley and Sons, 2001.

9 Whitaker S, Aw TC. Audit of pre-employment assessment by occupational health departments in the National Health Service. *Occupational Medicine* 1995; **45**(2): 75-80.

10 Hargreaves C. Screen test. *Occupational Health* 2006; **58**(7): 27-9.

11 Ballard J. Pre-employment health screening. Part 1: pre-employment questionnaires. *Occupational Health [at Work]* 2006; **3**(3): 18-25.

12 Kloss D. Pre-employment screening. Part 2: honesty, disability and knowledge. *Occupational Health [at Work]* 2006; **3**(3): 35-6.

13 Information Commissioner. Employment Practices Code (available at www.ico.gov.uk); 2005.

14 Smedley J, Dick F, Sadhra S. *Oxford Handbook of Occupational Health*. Oxford: Oxford University Press, 2007.

15 Faculty of Occupational Medicine. *Guidance on Ethics for Occupational Physicians*. London: FOM, 2006.

16 RCN. *Occupational Health Audit: A Practical Guide for Occupational Health Nurses*. London: RCN, 1999.

17 Agius RM. *Audit in Occupational Health:2. The Application of Audit to Occupational Health and Medicine* (available at www.agius.com/hew/audit/.hmt); 1995-2001.

18 Lewis J, Thornbory G. *Employment Law and Occupational Health: A Practical Handbook*. Oxford: Blackwell Publishing, 2006, p. 6.

19 NMC. *Record Keeping* (available at www.nmc-uk.org); 2007.

20 NMC. *The Code: Standards of Conduct, Performance and Ethics for Nurses and Midwives* (available at www.nmc-uk.org); 2007.

21 Butterworth C. Be a VIP - visible, informed and positive. *Occupational Health* 2008; **60(**8): 32-3.

22 HSE. *Health Surveillance at Work HSG61*. Bootle: HSE, 1999.

23 Wilson JMG, Junger G. Principles and practice of screening for disease. *WHO Chronicles* 1968; **22**(11): 4-73.

24 The Employment Equality (Age) Regulations 2006.

25 HSE. *Health Surveillance for Occupational Dermatitis G403* (available at www.hse.gov.uk/pubns/guidance/g403.pdf); 2006.

26 British Occupational Health Research Foundation. *Occupational Asthma: A Guide for Employers, Workers and Their Representatives* (available at www.bohrf.org.uk/content/asthma.htm); 2004.

27 HSE. *Colour Vision Examination* (available at www.hse.gov.uk/pubns/guidance/web03.pdf); 2005.

28 Control of Noise at Work Regulations 2005.

29 CBI/AXA. *At Work and Working Well? Absence and Labour Turnover Survey*. London: CBI/AXA, 2008.

30 Chartered Institute of Personnel and Development. *Annual Survey Report: Absence Management* (available at www.cipd.co.uk). London: CIPD, 2008.

31 Whitaker SC. The management of sickness absence. *Occupational and Environmental Medicines* 2001; **58**(6): 420-24.

32 Walters M. *One Stop Guide to Absence Management*. Surrey: Reed Business Information, 2005.

33 Advisory Conciliation and Arbitration Service. *Managing Attendance and Employee Turnover* (available at www.acas.org.uk); 2006.

34 Holford P, Nagle W, Rix D. Food for thought. *Occupational Health* 2008; **60**(6): 42-3.

35 Preeece R. OH needs to communicate effectively with GPs. *Occupational Health* 2008; **60**(8): 10.

36 Waddell G, Burton AK. *Concepts of Rehabilitation for the Management of Common Health Problems.* London: TSO, 2004.

37 Vocational Rehabilitation Association. *Standards of Practice.* London: VRA, 2007.

38 Waddell G, Burton AK. *Is Work Good for your Health and Wellbeing?* London: TSO, 2006.

39 Hughes V, ed. *Tolley's Guide to Employee Rehabilitation.* London: Lexis Nexis, 2004.

40 Black C. *Working for a Healthier Tomorrow: A Review of the Health of Britain's Working Age Population* (available at www.workingforhealth.gov.uk); 2008.

41 *Working for Health* (available at www.workingforhealth.gov.uk); 2008.

Chapter 9

Education and Continuing Professional Development of Public Health Nurses

Rebecca Elliott

Learning objectives

After reading this chapter you will be able to:

- Identify how education and continuing professional development contributes to improving quality of practice
- Appreciate regulatory need to maintain professional registration
- Be able to record learning events in order to maintain registration
- Recognise how learning styles influence learning and development
- Recognise the differences in academic levels of study in which they may participate in
- Utilise reflection throughout learning and professional development

Introduction

> The Kaleidoscope offers a metaphor – the symmetry, brilliance and ever-moving views of the professions. Each turn of the disk brings a new image, renewed vision and refreshment [1].

This description of Chaska of the developing nursing profession in the 1990s captured the need for education and continuing professional development (CPD) for the nurses to deal with the changing practice arena. This has still not changed in the twenty-first century as with every different view within that kaleidoscope of our roles, nurses need the knowledge and skills to make sense of what they see in practice and provide the expected outcomes of holistic health improvement. This is especially pertinent for the specialist community public health nurse as we strive to assist populations in managing these changing images within their community environments and influence the patterns of health that become visible. Public health nurses need to have the knowledge and skills to influence the way the light refracts upon the crystals within the kaleidoscope of our changing environment. Education and CPD to the learner should be as exciting as a child looking through a kaleidoscope. The practitioner can demonstrate learning and enhancing practice in a variety of ways and the portfolio of practice is becoming the accepted method for practitioners to demonstrate and record their competence through professional development [2]. This chapter will enable you as a practitioner to be able to recognise when learning takes place and that all learning is not a formal activity.

Professional development for nurses has changed throughout the centuries influenced by different cultures, society, politics, economical factors and great nursing leaders [3]. There continues to be much debate around the professionalisation of the nurse and although there is no time to discuss this area within this chapter, this aspect is worthy of further reading in understanding where you are today in your career [4]. CPD is the maintenance, improvement and broadening knowledge with the development of personal qualities in order to effectively carry out one's duties.

In 2000, the government set out their plans for improving the education, training and professional development of health and social care staff [5]. The document *Working Together, Learning Together: A Framework for Lifelong Learning* [6] set out the core vision for implementing the government's plans. This document discusses reasons as to why as a professional, we need to be continuously developing in relation to practice and at the heart of the vision lies the belief that professional development should be valued by everyone working in health and social care. Although not all learning is done formally, learning programmes should be based on individual needs and rooted in practice. Access to education, training and development should be flexible and show diversity with no discrimination in terms of age, sex, gender, ethnicity with accessibility for part-time workers and for all geographical areas. Accreditation should be awarded wherever possible, recorded, valued and recognised. Whenever practical, learning should be in shared groups and with different professions. CPD refers to any lifelong learning activities undertaken once qualified or in a chosen career.

The motivation to undertake professional development through formal education may be varied but there will always be key principles involved albeit in varying degrees:

- To maintain professional registration
- Personal development
- The quest to improve standards in practice
- Protection against litigation

Self-awareness is an important aspect of CPD. Self-awareness through reflection is fundamental to being able to assess the need for new knowledge, identify the learning which has taken place; problem solving in areas of practice to achieve the required outcomes and for the recall of evaluating the effectiveness of any health intervention undertaken. The clinical governance framework introduced in the White paper *The New NHS: Modern, Dependable* [7] joined a range of initiatives aimed at improving practice which included reflective practice together with evidence-based practice to ensure clinical effectiveness. This is also clearly defined in the nurse's professional code of practice [8], where it says that nurses should provide the best standard of care at all times using best available practice and keep one's knowledge and skills up to date. Reflection will be addressed in more detail later in this chapter.

Education and CPD in relation to professional registration

The Nursing and Midwifery Council (NMC) in the United Kingdom has the core function of setting standards for education, training, conduct and performance of nurses and midwives. By ensuring these standards are maintained, the NMC protects the safety of the public [9] (see Chapter 2). It is pertinent to recognise the role of the NMC in influencing the educational needs for the developing role of the nurse especially the public health nurse role. The emergence of the nurse prescriber to independent prescriber exemplifies this as just one of many examples of the political influences on health provision utilising limited resources for effective delivery of health care with the user in mind that has required regulatory changes to keep up with the developments. The school nurse may identify a priority need to prescribe in order to meet the needs of their populations [10]. Nurse prescribing offers school nurses the opportunity to make a difference to the health of teenagers who often present with multiple health-damaging behaviours [11]. The changes in regulation to enable practitioners to meet the needs of their client groups emphasises the need for education and CPD. As the NHS celebrates 60 years in existence the Darzi review for NHS reforms [12] continues to influence the need for CPD to fulfil the workforce expectations of this review.

Currently, the pathway-specific specialist public health nurse is registered on the third part of the nursing register [13]; however, as the Darzi [9] review states there is to be great emphasis on the prevention of ill health and maintenance of health within the NHS reforms and this equates to a high profile for the public health role of all nurses. Darzi [9] identified the following areas which require immediate steps in relation to public health:

- Primary Care Trusts will commission well-being services and prevention services in partnership with local authorities
- Services personalised to meet needs of local communities
- Working with voluntary and independent sector
- Coalition for better health
- Health of the workforce
- Primary and community care
- NICE
- Access for all practitioners to evidence-based information

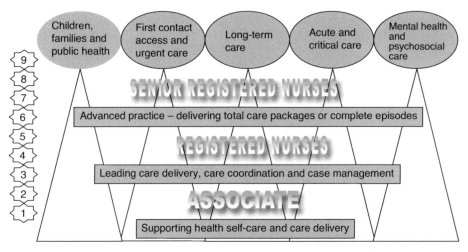

Figure 9.1 The model for nurse training: five proposed pathways (adapted from the DH [14].)

This will bring with it the need for changing workforce roles as the specialist public health practitioners alone on the third part of the register will not be able to fulfil the expected outcomes of this review. This has been partially addressed following the recent consultative review for post-registration nurse training [14]. The suggested model for training described five pathways in nursing which included a children, family and public health pathway (Figure 9.1). Note that within the proposed model of nursing pathways the agenda for change pay structure bandings have been utilised to demonstrate role competency descriptors.

Within the NHS, the agenda for change pay structure [15] works on the basis of knowledge, responsibility skills and effort needed for the job rather than a job title. It was a radical change to recognise the changing roles within the NHS from support workers (associate) to the advanced role. The agenda for change also had a real purpose to identify staff development needs during the personal development reviews and links closely to the knowledge and skills framework [16]. Recognising that although the NHS remains the main provider of health care within the UK this is changing and many PH nurses work outside the NHS. This is particularly true for OH specialists and in this case it will be market forces which determine pay bandings in relation to remuneration for services. School nurses also practice in private schools or social enterprises and so may health visitors. Although market forces may provide lucrative salaries, the practitioner would be well advised to enquire on offer of employment how CPD needs will be addressed within their new employment. As discussed later in the chapter this does not just relate to monies allocated for formal education, but also relates to time allocated to clinical supervision, evidence-based practice, and audit to enable reflection of experiences which enhances learning.

The response report [11] identified that further consultation through informed debate is needed in relation to how to present educational models for the PH nurse of the future. It is vital for education needs to be met for the health care workforce to perform effectively in public health, particularly with regards to health promotion in a multidisciplinary setting (see Figure 9.1) [11].

The White Paper *Trust, Assurance and Safety: The Regulation of Health Care Professionals in the 21st Century* [17] may very well have tremendous repercussions for the regulation and registration of PH nurses as the government states that they believe all professionals practicing in the same area should be subjected to the same standard of training, education and practice and this will involve the harmonisation of standards for the regulators. This paper also addresses the need for regulating health care support workers already referred to in a previous chapter, e.g. OH technicians. Current PH nurses and aspiring PH nurses need to be aware of these imminent changes and how they contribute to the overall goals of public health.

The role of the nurse may change in light of these political expectations. The current method of maintaining registration on the Nursing and Midwifery Register includes the requirement of CPD. Post-registration education and practice (PREP) [18] was first introduced in 1995 by the former UKCC (see Chapter 2). The NMC's latest version of PREP [15] includes the new rules relating to the re-registration of the specialist community public health nurse [10]. At re-registration every three years, nurses on whichever part of the register have to declare that they have complied with the PREP (CPD) standard [14]. The standard relates to the minimum amount of practice hours that needs to have been completed in a particular field of nursing and to the amount of CPD hours that needs to have been undertaken in the three years prior to re-registering (see Box 9.1).

Remember that any work you are involved with related to your role can be classed as practice hours. For example, this may include looking after children,

---

Box 9.1 The amount of practice hours required as adapted from *The PREP Handbook* [18]

Renewing your registration for	Practice hours required
Nursing	450
Midwifery	450
Nursing and Midwifery	900
Nursing and Specialist Community Health Nursing	450
Midwifery and Specialist Community Health Nursing	900
Nursing, Midwifery and Specialist Community Public Health Nursing	900

a disabled or elderly relative or friend. Helping at St Johns Ambulance or the Red Cross, accompanying a trip to Lourdes or anything which utilises your nursing skills paid or unpaid can contribute to the required practice hours. The remit of the standards for proficiency for the public health nurse is so broad that any work either paid or unpaid that influences the health and well-being of a community could be classed as practice. For example, working with the local cubs group on a safety project, lobbying the council for some improvement in services, or being a member of the parent-teacher association assisting in assessing the needs of the school children.

Activity 9.1

Take a few moments to refresh your knowledge of the NMC standards of proficiency for the SCPHN outlined in Chapter 2 and then make a list of further activities you can think of which would have a public health role and may count towards unpaid practice experience.

The PREP CPD standard also requires all registrants to undertake a minimum of 35 hours of learning activity in the three years prior to their re-registration and to maintain a professional portfolio. The NMC may ask to see a portfolio as part of their audit process. It is important to recognise that the form of learning activity undertaken can be varied, including both formal and informal activities, e.g. it may be a formal course with cost implications or informal where learning takes place through an experience which contributes to professional development for your role in public health. Indeed, you may not even be in paid employment whilst undertaking some learning-related activity which could count towards your CPD. This often causes confusion for some practitioners. CPD can be evidenced from any experience which contributes to their learning in relation to their practice.

Activity 9.2

Look back at the experiences you identified as being 'practice experience' in Activity 9.1. Take one and identify what you learnt from that experience. Did you identify any sharing and discussing information with your associates? Did you spend time web looking for information or journal/magazine articles?

The previous two exercises you have undertaken are exactly the type of information which needs to be recorded in the professional portfolio. There is no set format for a personal professional portfolio; however, any learning activity must inform your work role or plans for work in the future and it must help contribute to the best possible standard of practice possible (see Box 9.2).

Box 9.2   What should be included in a personal professional portfolio

- Record your normal place of work or experience
- Name the organisation you have been working for or identify if not working
- Brief description of your work role if not working, ensure you describe the learning activity or what you are claiming represents practice
- Record the date and briefly describe the nature of the learning activity, what did you do?
- Record the learning outcome you achieved and how this experience influenced your work. This section will include your personal views (reflections) on how the experience will influence the way you practice.

Case Study 9.1

It is breast cancer awareness month (http://www.breastcancercare. org.uk/content.php). So, I attended an informal networking learning lunch where a colleague was sharing her research undertaken a few years ago, relating to how scientists talk to lay people relating to possible causes of breast cancer. As a PH nurse with a health promotion role, I was interested in relating any new perspectives on how we can promote the health of women. The research involved interviewing and focus group discussions with the scientists involved in researching breast cancer. This included clinicians, toxicologists, policy makers and interested parties. The methodology included face-to-face interviews with prominent specialists in their fields and data from the focus groups using 'graffiti walls'.

Outcome - how did it relate to your work?

The results of the research identified a definite discourse in the opinions of the researchers; this in turn influences how public health policy and messages of health promotion are promoted to women. It made me think that this would be an excellent example to use with students in relation to how we use the evidence base for practice.

The methodology used for the research was interesting as I had never come across the use of graffiti walls where the members of the focus groups are asked to put comments under specific questions for their thoughts and feelings. I thought this was a very quick way to gain quality data on which to analyse a research question, one which I felt I could use in my work. I was also alerted to the feminine label attached to the 'pinkness' of breast cancer. Would this alienate some sufferers? Not all women may want to be associated with the 'Barbie doll' image and indeed breast cancer does not just affect the female gender.

The discussions made me think that, although death rates have been slashed by new drugs and early diagnosis, the incidence of breast cancer continues to rise. Research continues to be focused around cures not causes. Public health policy differs in the UK from the United States. I learned that some states have banned the use of certain substances in relation to breast cancer. Although the evidence may not be substantial some states work on the ethos of the precautionary principle where the evidence of harm rather than the definitive proof of harm prevail. Why is it that in the UK environmental causes are not taken seriously enough to warrant extensive research funding?

I will use knowledge from this new example of how 'business' and management of risk influences public health policy. Like the initiatives around smoking it had taken a long time to take action against the business empire, maybe in the future banning the use of some deodorants or use of hormones to feed livestock for consumption which even if not consumed can still enter the environment may be achieved. My future health promotion lectures will certainly include details of the 'precautionary principle' when discussing public policy.

Personal development

You may have difficulty in deciding what to do in relation to education and professional development at whatever stage your career is at. Everybody pursuing a learning activity, including any formal course for professional development, needs to be aware what is motivating them. The personal driving forces to achieve will certainly influence the outcome, successful or otherwise. Motivation can come from a variety of sources. Maslow [19], when discussing motivation and our drive to succeed, believed that there is a hierarchy of human needs from physical needs to spiritual self-actualisation (see Chapter 3). Innate personal traits to succeed will also be influenced by the society in which we live in; for example, we may need to drink but do we want water or wine? Likewise, the organisations in which we work can also influence our motivation to undertake CPD. The learning organisation will encourage, praise and reward those individuals willing to go beyond the boundaries to develop safe and effective practice [20]. It is important for you to identify all the different factors so you can also be aware of the barriers and challenges you may face and prepare for them. This would increase your chances of success in any goal you aim for. Case study 9.2 is a typical example of how nurses, who have embraced some form of education, develop their practice.

> **Case Study 9.2**
>
> When I started my nursing career as an SEN in 1979, I could never have envisaged either wanting or needing to undertake study to degree level. By 1998, the world of nursing was a very different place and I found myself having to embark on a degree course in OH in order to continue to practice this speciality. I did not want to do it and at the time I could not see the point of doing it, how wrong you can be? Obtaining my degree has been akin to a lottery win as far as its effect on my career. I have gained knowledge and confidence and as a result of this I have had the courage to develop my practice in very innovative ways. Studying for my degree inspired a passion within me that I did not know existed. I have gone on to study at masters level, I have had my work published and I have developed systems of working within OH that have been acknowledged by the HSE and the Employers Organisation. I am where I am today because of education and I would encourage all nurses to embrace the opportunity to open up their working lives through education.

Pedagogy and andragogy

Pedagogy is defined as the art, science and profession of teaching with andragogy being the term used for the teaching and training of adults [21]. Education and CPD for the PH nurse will be an andragogical experience and motivation influences the assumptions made about adult learners. It can be argued that to be successful in education one needs to be aware of these differences in education stances. Students describe a feeling of apprehension with some teaching styles (e.g. seminar work or presenting to groups). Self-awareness in personal motivation will give you the skill to identify which learning activity is best suited not just for your practice needs (knowledge and skills) but also for enjoyment of the learning experience. Read Case study 9.2 again; the reflections expressed note how the student's views changed during their educational experience from 'needing to know' in order to practice to having a life-centred orientation to learning, involving problem-solving and task-centred approaches in relation to developing practice.

Personal learning styles

CPD is also important for the health promotion role of the PH nurse. Personal learning styles influence the way we learn, they are the preferential modes in which a student likes to master learning, thinks or simply reacts in a learning situation. Honey and Mumford [22] defined four distinct learning styles or preferences: activist, pragmatist, theorist and reflector. They recommended

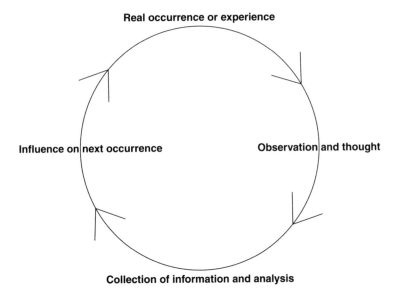

Figure 9.2 The learning cycle. (Adapted by Elliot.)

that in order to maximise your personal learning each learner ought to understand their learning style and seek out opportunities to learn using that style. This is important in our current society where demands are placed on us both professionally and socially as adult learners, forcing us to prioritise how we divide our time between home and work. Based upon the work of Kolb's [23] learning cycle (Figure 9.2) (discussed in Welsh and Swann [24]) Honey and Mumford [23] argue that identification of your preferred learning style will:

- Develop your learning skills and processes
- Broaden the type of experiences from which you can gain benefit
- Become smarter at getting a better fit between learning opportunities and the way you learn the best making learning easier and more enjoyable

E-learning
With e-learning expanding through the first decade of the twenty-first century it is important to recognise the process of learning that is taking place. In relation to professional practice for the PH nurse the outcome is for safe practice and quality practice development. E-learning is a quick, efficient and viable method to undertake continual professional development. Most structured courses will utilise e-learning and can be an integral part of any course. Known as 'learning objects', when used on the web, the expectation from students is to absorb information quickly via pictures, text or videos. However, learning is much more than receiving knowledge, it is about having the ability to reflect upon an experience, analyse the information and, from the learning, influence behaviour. Today, the web has moved from being a medium in which information was transmitted and consumed into being a platform from which content is

generated, shared, remixed and passed along. Individuals now interact and reflect on the web by having conversations and creating information (blogging). People no longer do need to be on formal courses to access various learning objects as e-learning can be an effective way to contribute towards CPD.

Online professional discussion groups are an ideal way to share information and to be guided by fellow professionals. One example of many offering this opportunity within the UK is JISCmail. JISCmail has the mission to facilitate knowledge sharing within the academic community using e-mail and the web, through provision, support and development of specialist mailing list-based services, enabling the delivery of high-quality and relevant content. JISCmail, or The National Academic Mailing list Service, is funded by JISC (www.jisc.ac.uk) to benefit learning, teaching and research. As with all aspects of practice the skill of the evidence-based practitioner is particularly pertinent with this technological revolution in the ability to understand and critique any evidence in the public domain.

Academic levels of study

The NMC has stated that a new framework for pre-registration training is to be developed and will be at the minimum level of a first degree. The curriculum content and delivery of the training is still at the consultative stage. Currently, the minimum level of entry to the third part of the nursing register as a specialist community public health nurse is to have completed a validated academic course at degree level. Many validated courses for entry onto the third part of the register offer courses at Post Graduate Diploma level. This gives the opportunity for the students to progress their academic development if they already have a first degree in a health-related subject [25]. It is important to note that not all forms of study used for CPD will carry academic credit and you need to check carefully, dependent on your personal requirements, as to which academic level any programme of study is awarded. This is also an important point to check in researching CPD requirement in relation to any recognised professional qualification required.

Academic level awards are assessed through attainment of learning objectives. These learning objectives are different dependent on the level of study undertaken. All Higher Education Institutions are quality assured to ensure their levels of study are equal in order for Credit Accumulation Transfer (CATS) [26]. The descriptors in Table 9.1 clearly show the different application of knowledge required for practice at various levels. These are also linked to agenda for change and knowledge for skills frameworks [12, 13].

European quality framework

The commission of the European Communities is working towards the European quality framework (EQF) for lifelong learning. In 1999, along with

Table 9.1 The different application of knowledge required at different levels.

Award	Level CATS	Descriptor
Diploma of Higher Education Foundation degrees [27]	1 and 2	Extends and re-enforces theoretical/practical aspects of knowledge
Degree (may be Hons)	1, 2 and 3	Demonstrates critical analysis and demonstrates ability in the manipulation and transfer of subject material to demonstrate a solid understanding of the issues in both theory and practice
Post Graduate Diploma (Masters)	M	Demostrates independent thought, synthesis of ideas and the generation of alternative views and information
Doctoral Degree	PhD	Original contribution to field of knowledge

28 European countries, the UK Government signed the Bologna Declaration, demonstrating a willingness to develop and cooperate in the European Higher (HE) Education Arena [28]. The education ministers agreed that there would be a common structure of HE across Europe by 2010. In 1999, it was agreed that all university qualifications would be transparent to employers and comparable. This was to increase student mobility across the European Union and work opportunities. The Bologna Declaration also affected vocational courses and the Tuning project is looking at the harmonisation of nursing courses including post-registration [29].

Cognitive skills

Cognitive skills (thinking skills) are assessed alongside practical skills for validated courses by the NMC, examples of cognitive skills are:

- Knowledge
- Comprehension
- Application
- Analysis
- Synthesis
- Evaluation

It is clear that for these cognitive skills to be addressed they must be parallel to practical skills. The NMC validated courses for entry to the SCPHN register require 50% theory and 50% practice. Quality and standards of the courses are reviewed regularly and aim to ensure students completing these courses are fit to practice. One of the incentives for using a portfolio within professional practice is to link the theory to practice and to be able to assess academic level [30].

SCPH nurses are expected to be able to consider broader issues that influence the health and well-being of their populations. This involves being able to identify health indicators such as poverty, social inequity based on gender, ethnicity, race, sexual orientation, physical and mental ability and other indicators leading to inequality of health particularly that of a political nature [31] (see Chapter 2). This is why the education of PH nurses needs to be at degree level ensuring competency in cognitive skills of problem solving resulting in political competence, action and activism to influence practice rather than just in clinical skills.

The need for evidence-based practice

Within the complex and rapidly changing environment for SCPHN, it is essential that practice is informed by the best available evidence. This commitment is reflected in the standards of proficiency. It includes searching the evidence base, analysing, critiquing, using research and other forms of evidence in practice, and disseminating research findings and adapting practice where necessary. The ability to synthesise new knowledge into practice, applying it to all areas of work where it is relevant and likely to be effective, must be reflected in all we do.

PH nurses need the knowledge and skills to be able to identify the reliability and validity of any information to develop, implement, evaluate and improve practice on the basis of any research. These cognitive skills which are then demonstrated in competent practice include being able to:

- Evaluate existing evidence and effectively apply to practice
- Appraise a range of research methods and other forms of generating evidence
- Demonstrate ability to utilise IT skills in databases, bibliographic packages and appreciate methods of data analysis
- Examine clinical issues from the students' practice, or that of others, using a systematic problem-solving approach
- Demonstrate knowledge of the sources and key concepts of evidence and how to assist clients in interpreting evidence

The standards of proficiency must, therefore, reflect a breadth of practice and of learning, at a level commensurate with the specialist nature of community public health nursing practice. This requires an ability to assess risk in complex situations; to develop effective relationships based on trust and openness; to work flexibly with other services in a range of settings; to deal with conflicting priorities and ambiguous situations; and knowing when to use different and sometimes contradictory theories and perspectives. In order to achieve this PH nurse needs to demonstrate critical thinking.

Critical thinking and reflective practice

It is not sufficient simply to have an experience in order to learn. Without reflecting upon this experience it may quickly be forgotten, or its learning potential lost. It is from the feelings and thoughts emerging from this reflection that generalisations or concepts can be generated. And it is generalisations that allow new situations to be tackled effectively [32].

All the previous discussions point to the need for proficient specialist nurse practitioners to demonstrate competency in critical thinking in order to practice competently and develop. So what does it mean to be critical? What does it mean to be a critical thinker in order to practice effectively and contribute to practice development as the standards state? A critical thinker never accepts what they have read or what they have experienced without further investigation. They are motivated and excited to probe and enquire 'why is that?' A critical thinker will want to know how that information came to be. In the case of any research, the methodologies will be critically reviewed. Was that the best research method to obtain the answer to the question under investigation? In the case of practice issues the question to be answered is 'why do we do that?' In the case of any experience we should be asking 'what can I learn from this?' Eventually, the critical thinker will be generating their own ideas as they investigate different phenomena to which they are exposed to and ultimately influence practice. In relation to learning through experience, a critical thinker will be analysing every angle of their exposure to a learning experience to explain why it happened as it did and how can we get it better next time? The learning experience may be as a result of a good experience or an experience leaving uncomfortable feelings.

Reflection and reflective learning are similar; reflective writing is capturing reflection and reflective practice is a term used in academic practice in many different ways. Reflection is a form of mental processing – like a form of thinking – that we use to fulfil a purpose or to achieve some anticipated outcome (learning to develop practice). It can be applied to relatively complicated or unstructured ideas for which there is not an obvious solution and is largely based on the further processing of knowledge and understanding and emotions that we already possess [33]. Reflective narrative is capturing these unstructured ideas, almost like in a movie to enable us to return to the event. Very often this is the narrative found in reflective journals used by many practitioners. It is the reflections within your portfolios that capture the learning and is the evidence of CPD as required for PREP [18].

Reflection is widely accepted as one of the main tools within any education to promote learning and critical analysis [32]. We tend to use reflection when we are trying to make sense of how diverse ideas fit together, when we are trying to relate new ideas to what we already know or when new ideas challenge what we already know (i.e. taking a deep approach to learning). Reflection is the process we use when working with material that is presented in an unstructured manner often trying to create order from chaos.

It is often useful to utilise a model of reflection to provide guidance of the process. Most of us will say we reflect all the time but may never have 'captured the evidence' of doing so. Some practitioners may favour a particular model to use within their profiles to document their learning and CPD. Models can be useful to guide us through the process particularly if a beginner.

Johns' [34] reflective cycle can be used to guide us through six stages of reflection:

- **Description:** What happened? What, where and when? Who did/said what, what did you do/read/see hear? In what order did things happen? What were the circumstances? What were you responsible for?
- **Feelings:** What were you thinking about? What was your initial gut reaction, and what does this tell you? Did your feelings change? What were you thinking?
- **Evaluation:** What was good or bad about the experience? What pleased, interested or was important to you? What made you unhappy? What difficulties were there? Who/what was unhelpful? Why? What needs improvement?
- **Analysis:** What sense can you make of the situation? Compare theory and practice. What similarities or differences are there between this experience and other experiences? Think about what actually happened. What choices did you make and what effect did they have?
- **Conclusion:** What else could you have done? What have you learnt for the future? What else could you have done?
- **Action plan:** If it arose again what would you do? What would you do next time?

Johns' model of reflection [34] was originally developed for nursing practitioners. Johns suggests that the 'Model for Structured Reflection' is a technique that is especially useful in the early stages of learning how to reflect. It is a model which offers guidance to look at the influencing factors within an experience to enable the practitioner to become reflexive, demonstrate critical analysis and create new knowledge:

Looking in:

- Find a space to focus on self
- Pay attention to your thoughts and emotions
- Write down these thoughts and emotions

Looking out:

- Write a description of the situation
- What issues seem significant?
- Aesthetics
- What was I trying to achieve?
  - Why did I respond as I did?
  - What were the consequences for me and others?
  - How were others feeling?
  - How did I know this?
- Personal
  - Why did I feel the way I did within this situation?
- Ethics
  - Did I act for the best?
- What factors were influencing me?
- What knowledge did or could have informed me?
- Reflexivity
  - How does this situation relate to previous experiences?
  - How could I have handled this better?
  - What would have been the consequences of alternative actions?
  - How do I feel now about the experience?
  - How can I support myself and others better in the future?

Clinical supervision and clinical governance

Johns [34] argues strongly of the benefits of reflecting within a group with the use of a facilitator. This philosophy can be seen in the clinical supervision models as a remit of clinical governance [35]. There are many definitions of clinical supervision; however, it is generally seen as the participation in regular reflection to provide professional support and enhance development. Clinical supervision is non-hierarchical and should be distinguished from management supervisions, performance appraisals and case load supervision such as child protection. It is not to be confused with any form of counselling or incident debriefing. The Department of Health states that in order to enhance the delivery of care nurses must participate in clinical supervision. Clinical supervision contributes to lifelong learning and is a clear demonstration of an individual exercising their responsibility under clinical governance [37]. Braine [38] discusses CPD as a process of lifelong learning that supports clinical governance by ensuring that skills and knowledge are developed and that areas of practice which require development can be identified through reflection. Not all PH nurses will be working within the NHS but the principles of clinical governance to health care professionals wherever they work. They are supported by the NMC and are good practice. The various models available need to be adapted to suit the work areas in which you practice. Three models of clinical supervision can be seen below.

Educative (formative)
- How to develop an understanding of skills and ability
- How to understand the client better
- How to develop awareness of reaction and reflection on interventions
- How to explore other ways of working

Supportive (restorative)
- Exploring the emotional reaction to pain, conflict and other feelings during patient care can reduce burn out

Managerial (normative)
- How to address quality issues
- How to ensure nurses work reach appropriate standards

PH nurses will be employed in a variety of work organisations both within and outside NHS then creativity is required in order to achieve the best opportunity to ensure clinical supervision takes place. The RCN recommends various ways to create opportunities for personal or peer clinical supervision [39]:

- Utilise local specialist interest groups (these may even be online forums)
- Meeting with nurses from other organisations (it is within the standards to register as a specialist community public health nurse to undertake a minimum three weeks alternative practice within the training programme, many students on qualification commit to continue this practice for support and bench-marking purposes)
- Consider the opportunities for supervision with other professionals (this will contribute to the multidisciplinary working remit for public health needs of the population group)
- Using formal facilitated group supervision
- Using personal colleagues on a one-to-one basis

Whichever model is utilised, clinical supervision is supported by the NMC and fits into the CPD requirements for PREP.

Below is a short extract from a student's reflection. This piece demonstrates how critical reflection can aid learning and move practice forward.

> ## Case Study 9.3
> The company was experiencing vast changes. The disbandment of local Human Resource departments in favour of a central shared service centre in another region left groups and individuals feeling vulnerable and disorientated.
>
> I analysed my feelings and what I was experiencing with this transition. I went from working within a team to an autonomous lone practitioner where I was pushing personal comfort boundaries and growing into

the role of a SCPHN OH. Similarly, groups and individuals were experiencing the similar dilemmas. Even more changes were thrust upon them as they were taking ownership of sickness absence management at a local management level. I identified change was a major issue here for all involved. I applied what was happening using Tuckman's model of group development. My role within the organisation was still forming. Line managers however were displaying characteristics of the storming phase where as a group they had become polarized and sub groups were forming which manifested as varying degrees of resistance to my efforts to improve the standard of the OH referral forms. Tuckman describes this as reactions to power distribution and some resistance to the task. Similarly, Lewin acknowledges such a status quo as an existing equilibrium and identifies how one has to unfreeze such an existing equilibrium to enable the moving on to a new point. Lewin describes further the dynamics of change identifying that it was often met with a force field of both driving and restraining forces. In my case a driving force had emerged at government and organisational level, which required a new way of conducting sickness absence management, and it was essential for line managers to take ownership of this to ensure success.

Boud and Walker discuss that the responsible professional needs to master the ability to learn from their experiences and more importantly translate that learning into applied action identifying how essential reflective skills have become for me in my journey to become a SCPHNOH.

Note how her style of reflection has moved beyond the immediate picture (the current system of sickness absence management referral to OH not working effectively, preventing her performing her role to an appropriate standard as a SCPHN). Her journal or diary entry for the day may well have included a description of what happened, factual, related to practice, perhaps even recording her feelings. These further reflections are seeking out explanations, the answers to why the referral process is not working. The practitioner is looking at other influences on the situation and finding meaning by linking the theory of Tuckman [40] and Lewin's [41] change management. This is demonstrating how there is a 'stepping back' from the events and actions which led to the different level of discourse. There is a sense of 'mulling about', discourse with self and an exploration of the role of self in events and actions. There is consideration of the qualities of judgements and possible alternatives for explaining and hypothesising. The reflection is analytical and integrative, linking factors and perspectives. This critical reflection has also evidenced an awareness of multiple perspectives with a sociopolitical context.

Using reflection the student practitioner was able to analyse the situation and identify a suitable course of action to successfully work within a changing environment.

Permission was granted to reproduce the above reflective writing, however, all practitioners need to be aware of their legal standing in relation to confidentiality and reflective practice. The RCN states that where clinical supervision is required in a contract of employment the records belong to the employer and could be used in a disciplinary procedure. If it is not part of the contract of employment then the practitioner holds the records and confidentiality can be maintained as per the code of practice. For this reason it is important for the practitioner to agree what is documented within clinical supervision.

Contributing to the CPD of self and others

The new code, standards of conduct, performance and ethics for nurses and midwives [42] specifically relates to our role of assisting in the professional development of colleagues in order to improve standards of care and to the requirement for our own professional development.

- You must facilitate students and colleagues to develop their competence
- You must be willing to share your skills and experience for the benefit of your colleagues
- You must deliver care based on the best available evidence or practice
- You must keep your knowledge and skills up to date throughout your working life
- You must take part in appropriate learning and practice activities that maintain and develop your competence and performance

The NMC supports practitioners through lifelong learning to enable them to practice in an environment which is constantly changing. In the field of PH as with all health professional roles it is imperative to develop professional knowledge and competence to cope with the demands of increasing technological advances in treatment, equipment and reorganisation of resources. The NMC recognises that newly qualified registrants on any part of the register need the support and guidance of a more experienced professional colleague as they find their feet in practice. This would also apply to those returning to practice after a break of five years or more. The NMC believes that newly registered nurses need a period of preceptorship (minimum period of four months) [43]. A preceptorship period is also required for newly qualified SCPH nurses.

Standards to support learning and assessment in practice are the nursing and midwifery standards for mentors, practice teachers and teachers [44]. All student SCPH nurses have to be assessed and supported in practice by a qualified practice teacher who is qualified in the same area of practice in which the student is studying. All current qualified practitioners have the opportunity to support students and contribute to the development and standards of the public health nursing workforce. Indeed, without the continued support from current practitioners the public health workforce would not develop.

The framework defines and describes the knowledge and skills nurses and midwives need to apply in practice when they support and assess students undertaking NMC-approved programmes. It is important to understand these standards in order to support students and colleagues. The developmental framework and underpinning principles of the standards have been designed to allow personal and professional development. The domains and outcomes enable nurses and midwives to plan and measure their achievement and progress. The framework allows practitioners to map their previous learning experiences to the new standards in order to readily identify their personal learning needs:

Stage 1 reflects the requirements of the code; standards of conduct, performance and ethics for nurses and midwives [44]. All nurses and midwives must meet this defined requirement in particular: 'you must, help students and others to develop their competencies'.

Stage 2 identifies the standards for mentors. This qualification is recorded on a local register of mentors and sign off mentors.

Stage 3 identifies the standards required of the practice teacher for assessing a SCPHN is fit to enter that part of the register. Some commissioners of education also require the specialist qualification programme to use a practice teacher for assessment, e.g. district nursing. This qualification is also recorded on a local register.

Stage 4 identifies the standard for a teacher of nursing and this is recordable with the NMC.

Figure 9.3 shows the stages, principles and domains of the standards to support learning and assessment in practice.

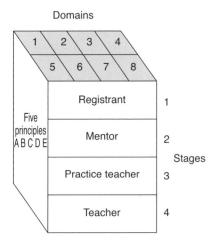

Figure 9.3 The stages, principles and domains of the standards to support learning and assessment in practice (adapted from NMC [14]).

Box 9.3 shows the NMC's stages, principles and domains of the standards required to support learning and assessment in practice.

> ## Box 9.3 The NMC stages, principles and domains of the standards to support learning and assessment in practice
>
> **Principle A** states that the nurses and midwives who make judgments need to be on the same part of the register or sub-register as that which the student is wanting to enter
>
> **Principle B** states that they must have developed their knowledge, skills and competency beyond that of initial registration through CPD either formal or informal
>
> **Principle C** states that they will hold an appropriate level of professional qualification to support and assess the students they mentor/teach (equal to or higher)
>
> **Principle D** requires that they have been prepared for their role
>
> **Principle E** states that those who have completed a teacher's qualification to NMC standards may record the qualification with the NMC.

The domains refer to the key areas of knowledge to which competencies have to be achieved in order to reach the differing stages.

The domains are:

(1) Establishing effective working relationships
(2) Facilitation of learning
(3) Assessment and accountability
(4) Evaluation of learning
(5) Create an environment for learning
(6) Context of practice
(7) Evidence-based practice
(8) Leadership

Due to the lack of qualified practice teachers in some pathways for the SCPHN (especially occupational health), the assessment of the specialist skills is done by a registrant and shared accountability with a qualified practice teacher is required for confirmation of overall proficiency to enter the third part of the register as a SCPHN [44].

Summary

To summarise, education and CPD is the responsibility of every nurse, midwife and SCPHN. However, because PH is growing at an astonishing speed due to public health need and the political drivers it is imperative that practicing professionals and those students of PH nursing contribute to the development of self and others following the philosophy of the multidisciplinary team for optimum benefit of resources and quality of service to the users.

In this climate of reduced resources it is evident that all opportunities for development need to be grasped and education does not always have a monetary cost. Any learning can be valued for CPD whether it is from watching a television programme, surfing the web or a discussion with colleagues. What does require the skill is to be able to reflect and identify the learning that has taken place; this skill can be learned and developed. Education for CPD should be as exciting to the professional as the kaleidoscope is to a child. In seeking for the different shapes and views, even creating the views, we strive to enhance the quality of our practice in public health.

References

1 Chaska N. *The Nursing Profession – Turning Points*. St Louis: Mosby, 1990.
2 Timmins F. *Making Sense of Portfolios*: A Guide for Nursing Studies. Maidenhead, UK: Open University Press, 2008.
3 McGann S. *The Battle of the Nurses*. London: Scutari Press, 1992.
4 Hart C. *Nurses and Politics – The Impact of Power and Influence*. Basingstoke: Palgrave Macmillan, 2004.
5 DH. *The NHS Plan: A Plan for Investment, a Plan for Reform*. London: HMSO, 2000.
6 DH. *Working Together, Learning Together: A Framework for Lifelong Learning*. London: HMSO, 2001.
7 DH. *The New NHS: Modern, Dependable*. London: HMSO, 1997.
8 NMC. *The Code: Standards of Conduct, Performance and Ethics for Nurses and Midwives*. London: NMC Publications, 2008.
9 NMC. *The Nursing and Midwifery Council* (available at http://www.nmc-uk.org/aSection.aspx?SectionID=5); 2008. Accessed August 2008.
10 DH. *Every Child Matters, Change for Children Department for Education and Skills*. London: HMSO, 2006.
11 Day P. School nurse independent prescribing in practice. *British Journal of School Nursing* 2007; **2**(6): 267–71.
12 DH. *NHS the Next Stage Review – High Quality Care for All, NHS Reforms* (available at www.dh.gov.uk). Norwich: TSO, 2008.
13 NMC. *Standards of Proficiency for Specialist Community Public Health Nurses* (available at www.nmc-uk.org). London: NMC, 2004. Accessed July 2008.
14 DH. *Towards a Framework for Post Registration Nursing Careers: Consultation Response Report* (available at http://www.dh.gov.uk/en/Consultations/Responsestoconsultations/DH_086465); 2008.
15 DH. *Agenda for Change – The final Agreement* (available at http://www.dh.gov.uk/en/Publicationsandstatistics/Publications/PublicationsPolicyAndGuidance/DH_4095943); 2004. Accessed August 2008.
16 DH. *The Knowledge and Skills Framework (NHS KSF) and the Development Review Process*. London: HMSO, 2004.
17 UK Government. *Trust, Assurance and Safety: The Regulation of Health Care Professionals in the 21st Century* (available at http://www.official-documents.gov.uk/document/cm70/7013/7013.pdf). London: HMSO, 2007. Accessed August 2008.

18 NMC. *The PREP Handbook* (available at http://www.nmc-uk.org/aFrame-Display.aspx?DocumentID=4340); 2008.

19 Maslow A. *Motivation and Personality*. New York: Harper, 1954.

20 Pettinger R. *The Learning Organisation*. New York: John Wiley and Sons.

21 Quinn F, Hughes S. *Quinns Principles and Practice of Nurse Education*. Cheltenham: UK: Nelson Thornes, 2007.

22 Honey P, Mumford A. *The Manual of Learning Styles*, 3rd edn. Maidenhead: Peter Honey, 1992.

23 Kolb DA. Experiential learning: experience as the source of the learning and development. In: Welsh I, Swann C, eds. *Partners in Learning – A Guide to Support and Assessment in Nurse Education*. Abingdon: Radcliffe Medical Press, 2002.

24 Welsh I, Swann C. *Partners in Learning – A Guide to Support and Assessment in Nurse Education*. Radcliffe, UK: Prentice Hall, 2002.

25 Association of Occupational Health Educators (available at www.aohne.org.uk); 2009

26 Quality Assurance Agency for Higher Education (available at www.qaa.ac.uk); 2009

27 QAA. *Benchmark for Foundation Degrees*. London: TSO, 2002.

28 Editorial. *Education in Chemistry* 2005; **43**(2): 30.

29 Longley M, Shaw C, Dolan G. *Nursing Towards 2015*. London: Nursing and Midwifery Council, 2007.

30 Endacott R, Jasper M, McMullan M, Miller C, Pankhurst P, Scholes J, et al. Portfolios and assessment of competence: a review of the literature. *Journal of Advanced Nursing* 2003; **41**(3): 283-94.

31 Rideout E. *Transforming Nurse Education through Problem Based Nursing*. London: Jones and Bartlett, 2001.

32 Gibbs G. *Learning by Doing: A Guide to Teaching Methods*. Oxford: Oxford University Press, 1988.

33 Moon J. *Reflection in Learning and Professional Development*. London: Routledge Falmer, 1999.

34 Johns C. *Becoming a Reflective Practitioner: A Reflective and Holistic Approach to Clinical Nursing, Practice Development and Clinical Supervision*. Oxford: Blackwell Science, 2000.

35 DH. *Clinical Governance in the New NHS*. London: HMSO, 1999.

36 DH. *Public Health and Clinical Quality: Clinical Governance*. London: DH, 2002.

37 Butterworth T, Woods D. *Clinical Supervision and Clinical Governance: A Briefing Paper*. Manchester: University of Manchester, 1999.

38 Braine ME. Clinical governance applying theory to practice. *Nursing Standard* 2006; **20**: 56-65.

39 Royal College of Nursing. *Clinical Supervision for Occupational Health Nurses*. London: RCN, 2003.

40 Tuckman B. Effective working groups. In: Pettinger R, ed. *Mastering Organisational Behaviour*. Basingstoke, UK: Macmillan, 2000.

41 Lewin K. *Field Theory in Social Science*. New York: Harper.

42 NMC. *The Code, Standards of Conduct, Performance and Ethics for Nurses and Midwives* (available at www.nmc-uk.org). London: NMC, 2008.

43 NMC. *Supporting Nurses and Midwives through Life Long Learning*. London: NMC, 2002.

44 NMC. *Standards to Support Learning and Assessment in Practice*, 2nd edn. (available at www.nmc-org.uk). London: NMC, 2008.

Appendix

Public health resources

Public health organisations

The Joseph Rowntree Foundation: www.jrf.org.uk
West Midland Public Health Observatory: www.wmpho.org.uk
London Health Observatory: www.lho.org.uk
The World Bank: www.worldbank.org
Medecins Sans Frontieres: www.msf.org/
The Kings Fund: www.kingsfund.org.uk
World Health Organization: www.who.int/en/

Public health organisations related to government

Department for Children, Schools and Families: www.everychildmatters.gov.uk/
  health/schoolnurses/
Health Protection Agency: www.hpa.org.uk
Working for Health: www.workingforhealth.gov.uk
The Skills for Health Agency: www.skillsforhealth.org.uk/page/competences
Department of Health: www.dh.gov.uk
Health Development Agency: www.nice.org.uk
Quality Assurance Agency and Department of Health: www.qaa.ac.uk/reviews
Advisory, Conciliation and Arbitration Service (ACAS): www.acas.org.uk
Age Positive: www.agepositive.gov.uk
Health and Safety Executive: www.hse.gov.uk
UK National Screening Committee: www.nsc.nhs.uk
National Travel Health Network and Centre: www.nathnac.org
The Information Commissioner (regarding the Data Protection Act): www.
  ico.gov.uk
The Equality and Human Rights Commission: www.equalityhumanrights.com

Professional organisations related to public health

The Royal College of Nursing: www.rcn.org.uk
The Community Practitioners and Health Visitors Association: www.amicus-
  cphva.org
The Association of Occupational Health Nurse Practitioners: www.AOHNP.co.uk
United Kingdom Standing Conference on Health Visitor Education: www.uksc.org
The Association of Occupational Health Nurse Educators: www.aohne.org.uk
The School and Public Health Nurses Association: www.saphna-professionals.org
Public Health: www.publichealth.com

Faculty of Public Health: www.fphm.org.uk
British Occupational Health Research Foundation: www.bohrf.org.uk
International Council of Nurses: www.ICN.ch
Faculty of Occupational Medicine: www.facomen.ac.uk
Institute of Occupational Safety and Health: www.iosh.co.uk
The Ergonomics Society: www.ergonomics.org.uk
British Occupational Hygiene Society: www.bohs.org
International Hygiene Association: www.ioha.net
British Occupational Health Research Foundation: www.bohrf.org.uk
Case Management Society: www.cmsuk.org
NHS Plus: www.nhsplus.nhs.uk

Recommended reading on public health

Beaglehole R, ed. *Global Public Health: A New Era*. Oxford: Oxford University Press, 2003.

Beaglehole R, Bonita R, Horton R, Adams O, McKee M. Public health in the new era: improving health through collective action. *Lancet* 2004; **363**: 2084-6.

Davey B, Gray A, Seale C, eds. *Health and Disease: A Reader*, 3rd edn. Buckingham: Open University Press, 2001.

Detels R, McEwen J, Beaglehole R, Tanaka H, eds. *Oxford Textbook of Public Health*, 4th edn. Oxford: Oxford University Press, 2002.

Evans R, Barer M, Marmor T, eds. *Why Are Some People Healthy and Others Not?* Piscataway, MD: Aldine Transacations, 1994.

Last JM. *A Dictionary of Epidemiology*, 4th edn. Oxford/New York: Oxford University Press, 2001.

McKee M, Garner P, Stott R, eds. *International Co-operation and Health*. Oxford: Oxford University Press, 2001.

Pencheon D, Guest C, Melzer D, Gray M, eds. *Oxford Handbook of Public Health Practice*. Oxford: Oxford University Press, 2001.

Rose G. *The Strategy of Preventive Medicine*. Oxford: Oxford University Press, 1992.

Index

Maria Henderson Library
Gartnavel Royal Hospital
Glasgow G12 0XH Scotland